Prayers
for
DIFFICULT
TIMES

Cancer

© 2017 by Barbour Publishing, Inc.

Print ISBN 978-1-68322-318-4

eBook Editions:
Adobe Digital Edition (.epub) 978-1-68322-523-2
Kindle and MobiPocket Edition (.prc) 978-1-68322-524-9

All rights reserved. No part of this publication may be reproduced or transmitted for commercial purposes, except for brief quotations in printed reviews, without written permission of the publisher.

Churches and other noncommercial interests may reproduce portions of this book without the express written permission of Barbour Publishing, provided that the text does not exceed 500 words or 5 percent of the entire book, whichever is less, and that the text is not material quoted from another publisher. When reproducing text from this book, include the following credit line: "From *Prayers for Difficult Times: Cancer*, published by Barbour Publishing, Inc. Used by permission."

Scripture quotations marked KJV are taken from the King James Version of the Bible.

Scripture quotations marked NIV are taken from the HOLY BIBLE, NEW INTERNATIONAL VERSION®. NIV®. Copyright © 1973, 1978, 1984, 2011 by Biblica, Inc.™ Used by permission. All rights reserved worldwide.

Scripture quotations marked MSG are from THE MESSAGE. Copyright © by Eugene H. Peterson 1993, 1994, 1995, 1996, 2000, 2001, 2002. Used by permission of NavPress Publishing Group.

Scripture quotations marked NLT are taken from the Holy Bible. New Living Translation copyright© 1996, 2004, 2015 by Tyndale House Foundation. Used by permission of Tyndale House Publishers, Inc. Carol Stream, Illinois 60188. All rights reserved.

Scripture quotations marked NASB are taken from the New American Standard Bible, © 1960, 1962, 1963, 1968, 1971, 1972, 1973, 1975, 1977, 1995 by The Lockman Foundation. Used by permission.

Published by Barbour Books, an imprint of Barbour Publishing, Inc., P.O. Box 719, Uhrichsville, Ohio 44683, www.barbourbooks.com

Our mission is to publish and distribute inspirational products offering exceptional value and biblical encouragement to the masses.

Member of the
Evangelical Christian
Publishers Association

Printed in the United States of America.

Prayers
for
DIFFICULT
TIMES

Cancer

Ellyn Sanna

BARBOUR BOOKS
An Imprint of Barbour Publishing, Inc.

Contents

Introduction 7
Something's Wrong 8
Fearing the Worst. 10
Waiting for Answers. 12
Diagnosis 15
Terror 18
Denial. 23
Bargaining with God 26
Anger 28
Grief. 32
Why Me? 36
Acceptance 39
Feelings of Doubt. 42
Prayers for My Friends. 46
Prayers for My Family 49
Prayers for My Spouse 52
Prayers for My Children. 55
Prayers for My Medical Team 58
Physical Pain 61
Emotional and Spiritual Pain. 65
Isolation and Loneliness. 68
Anxiety. 72
Help Me Relax, Lord! 76
Praise in the Midst of the Worst 80
When Others Don't Know What to Say 84
When It's Time to Fight 88
Feeling Bad Isn't Giving Up. 92

Surgery 95
Will I Ever Feel Normal Again? 100
When All Seems Hopeless. 103
When I Feel Helpless. 107
Recovery from Surgery. 111
Chemotherapy 114
Radiation 116
Dealing with the Side Effects. 119
Physical Weakness 122
Emotional and Spiritual Weakness. 125
Crying Out to God 128
Shame. 132
Asking Others for Help 136
Taking Care of Myself 140
Loving My Body 144
God's Promises. 148
Physical Healing. 154
Emotional Healing. 158
Spiritual Healing 162
Peace. 166
Hope. 171
Joy. 176
Love 181
Life. 186

Introduction

And the Holy Spirit helps us in our weakness. . . .
The Holy Spirit prays for us with groanings
that cannot be expressed in words.
ROMANS 8:26 NLT

∾

*W*hen the threat of cancer falls over our own lives, we feel sick with fear—but we can also begin to rely on God's presence in new ways. We realize that constant prayer is the only way to gain the strength we need. Prayer won't bring instant physical healing, but it seasons our hearts, making them able to bear things we never thought we could. We learn to surrender everything to God. Like Jesus in the garden of Gethsemane, we pray that we and our loved ones be spared this terrible thing—but like Jesus, we also learn to pray, "Not my will, Father, but Yours."

In moments of crisis, it's hard to know how to pray. These "prayer starters" are intended to be launchpads for your heart's cries. Many of them come from the Word, claiming God's promises of healing and victory. Use them to get your prayers started—and then keep going. And don't hesitate to simply pray with "groanings that cannot be expressed in words." God will understand.

Something's Wrong

Jesus spoke to them at once. "Don't be afraid,"
he said. "Take courage! I am here!"
MARK 6:50 NLT

∾

*C*aught in heavy winds at sea, the disciples look
out in the darkness and see the shape of a man
coming toward them. They're not sure what's going
on, but they sense that something's wrong—and
they're terrified. But then they hear a familiar voice
calling to them. At the very moment when they're
most afraid, they find themselves in the presence
of the Lord. Then Jesus climbs into the boat with
them, and the winds die down.

Facing the threat of cancer is a little like
what the disciples experienced. We're not sure
what's coming toward us—and we're terrified.
But Jesus calls to us, saying, "Don't be scared. I'm
here." He climbs into the situation with us—and
the winds die down. No matter what comes next,
He will be with us.

I'm not sure what's wrong, God. I'm not even sure
if anything *is* wrong. Maybe it will all prove to be
a false alarm. But whatever happens, don't leave
me. Stay close by. I can't do this without You.

Jesus, You know how scared I feel about this
situation. I want to be like Peter, though—brave
enough to even walk on water if that's what You
ask of me. I've never been in a situation quite like
this before, and everything inside me is saying it's
not right. But You can empower me to do things
I never thought I could. Help me keep my eyes
fixed on You so I won't sink and be overwhelmed.

Fearing the Worst

You will live in constant suspense, filled with dread both night and day, never sure of your life. In the morning you will say, "If only it were evening!" and in the evening, "If only it were morning!"— because of the terror that will fill your hearts.

DEUTERONOMY 28:66–67 NIV

∞

*W*hen we face the threat of cancer, our minds toss back and forth between hope and dread. We feel sick from the suspense—and there's no relief from these feelings. No one can say anything to take them away, and no matter what we're doing, they're always there, lurking at the back of our minds. When fear is constant, then constant prayer is the only way to cope. "If you can worry," Rick Warren wrote, "you can meditate, for worry is negative meditation."

Each time you feel that nagging, sick sense of dread, let it be a reminder to turn your attention to God in prayer. Let your fear be the voice of God calling to you.

My thoughts can find nowhere to rest, Lord.
When I'm working, I wish I were free to do
nothing but worry. Then when I'm not working,
I long for something to distract me. I want to
be with people—and then I just want to be
alone. The sense of suspense, the anxiety that
my worst fears will become reality, feels like
something inside me, gnawing on my insides.
O God, please help me!

Is that You, God? Are You here with me?
Come closer, I beg You. Let me feel Your hand.
Wrap me up in Your love. Take this terrible
fear from me, I pray.

I can't seem to make the fear go away—
so I'll give it to You. Please take it into
Your hands. Thank You, heavenly Father,
that You can use even fear to Your glory.

Waiting for Answers

*Wait for the LORD; be strong and
take heart and wait for the LORD.*
PSALM 27:14 NIV

∞

*O*nce all the tests have been done, there's
nothing left to do until we get the results. Will
it be good news—or bad? All we can do is wait.
We wish we could *do* something—but there's
nothing we can do to change the results. We feel
completely helpless.

Millennia ago, the psalmist experienced these
same emotions, and he reminded himself to "be
strong and take heart." What's more, he turned
around the situation, so that instead of waiting
for the world to hand him an end to his pain, he
shifted his attention to God—and then he was
waiting for his Lord.

Don't panic if darkness seems to hide God's
presence from you. Just wait for Him. In that
moment when you get your answers, God will be
there, too.

Beloved God, I'm waiting for You. Be real to me today. Make Your presence known to me. In the midst of my worry, may I see You so clearly that You drive away all other thoughts.

Give peace, I pray, to all the others who are worrying and waiting with me. Lead us all through this journey, singing songs of hope. Quiet our souls, quell our fears, and fill us with Your everlasting love.

Lord Jesus, when I lie in bed, unable to sleep because of the fear that grips my mind, may I feel You with me. May the peace of Your presence lie over me like a blanket. Remind me of all the ways You've helped me in the past. Help me dwell on those things rather than my anxiety.

Hold me close at this time of uncertainty, dear Lord. Remind me of Your promises. Sharpen my ears so that I hear Your Spirit whispering words of love. Quiet my mind so I can rest while I wait.

Let prayer be my strong lifeline,
tying me to the One who will never move,
regardless of what the future holds.

Remind me to smile today, Jesus. Let me not be so preoccupied that I miss out on the blessings You are still sending my way, even now.

Help me, loving God, to live one moment at a time. Give me strength to trust that no matter what comes, You do all things well. I surrender to Your will.

Diagnosis

They will have no fear of bad news;
their hearts are steadfast, trusting in the Lord.
PSALM 112:7 NIV

∞

*N*ow we know. The thing we feared most has
been confirmed. This is our new reality, a reality
that forces us to step back from the life we've been
living up until now. Suddenly, everything that
seemed so important—our endless to-do lists,
our small worries and preoccupations—has fallen
away, leaving an emptiness that's filled only with
the enormous, looming shape of cancer.

But take a deep breath. This diagnosis is not
a death sentence. Life still lies ahead, life in this
world and eternal life as well. And God is with us
here, in this new reality. He has things to teach us
if we are willing to learn. He even has ways He
wants to use us. As we trust in Him, He will give
us a new ministry, right here, right now—a new
way of carrying His love into the world.

Father, I want to trust You—but I feel
too wobbly to be "steadfast."
Please steady my heart and mind.

Jesus, on the night before Your death, You must
have felt a little like this—sick with anxiety,
terrified of the pain and death that had drawn
so near. I know You understand. Please use
this time to draw me closer to You.

Be with us, Lord, as my family and I
go through this time. May we not
be too scared to hear Your voice.

I know that we'll have to make many decisions
in the days ahead. We'll have to think about
treatment plans and what they will mean. We'll
also need to sort out all the ordinary business
of life—how this diagnosis will affect jobs
and family and our daily lives. It all seems so
overwhelming, especially right now. Draw me
closer to Your heart, dear Lord. I know that
when my heart is close to Yours, I will be better
able to deal with whatever comes next.

∞

Remind me, God, that this diagnosis affects not
only me but others as well. Help me be sensitive
to their needs. Use me as You see fit to speak Your
words of wisdom and comfort.

Terror

I am so bewildered I cannot hear, so terrified I cannot see.
My mind reels, horror overwhelms me.
ISAIAH 21:3–4 NASB

*F*ear is a normal and healthy biological reaction that alerts us to danger. By flooding our bodies with adrenaline, making our heartbeat increase and our breath come faster, fear was designed to prepare our bodies either to run away or take action. But when facing the reality of cancer, we can do neither of those things. We can't run away; we don't know how to take action. We feel helpless. We find ourselves frozen with terror—unable to hear, see, speak, or think.

That reaction is normal. As we move forward on this new path, the terror will retreat. But for now, simply know that God is still present. He is still our refuge. He is big enough to hold our fear, and He will never leave us.

You are my light and salvation, Lord.
You are my stronghold, so why should I
fear anything—even cancer? (Psalm 27:1).

∞

You are with me, Lord, so I won't be afraid.
What can cancer do to me when I have You?
(Psalm 118:6).

∞

You didn't give me a terrified spirit, God,
but a spirit of power, of love, and of
self-discipline (2 Timothy 1:7).

Send Your angel to encamp around me,
loving Lord. Deliver me (Psalm 34:7).

∞

Heavenly Father, I know You don't want me to
be in bondage to fear. And because Your Spirit
has adopted me, I can cry, "Daddy! Father"—
and I know You'll hear me! (Romans 8:15).

∞

Help me hear Your voice saying to me,
"Fear not, for I have redeemed you; I have
called you by name; you are Mine" (Isaiah 43:1).

Lord, You are my light and my salvation. Whom shall I fear? You are the strength of my life. Of whom shall I be afraid? When my enemies attack me, they'll stumble and fall. Though an entire army of fears comes against me, my heart will be strong. Even facing the reality of cancer, I can be confident in You, because I ask You for only one thing: that I may dwell in Your house all the days of my life, seeing Your beauty. For I know that now, in this time of trouble, You will hide me in Your pavilion. You'll tuck me away in a secret nook inside Your tabernacle; You'll set me on a rock where I'll be safe, where I can lift up my head and see beyond this illness. And that's why, Lord, I sing to You with joy— even now! (Psalm 27:1–6).

When we heard the diagnosis, our hearts melted in fear and everyone's courage failed. But we know that the Lord our God is God in heaven above and on the earth below. So I pray, dear Lord, that You will show kindness to my family. Give me confidence that You will be with us all—parents, grandparents, children, brothers, and sisters—and all who care about us—and that You will save us from death (Joshua 2:11–12).

Jesus, I hear Your voice telling me not to be afraid. "Look!" You say. "I'll care for everyone who travels with you on this journey. So take courage." I believe You, Jesus. I trust that it will happen just as You say (Acts 27:24–25).

Denial

Ye have purified your souls in
obeying the truth through the Spirit.
1 PETER 1:22 KJV

∞

*R*efusing to acknowledge that something is
wrong is a normal way to cope with anything
that puts our sense of control at risk—including
a serious illness that threatens ourselves or those
we love. A short period of denial can be helpful
because it gives us time to absorb this new reality
at a pace that won't send us into a tailspin.

But we can't linger in denial. Instead, we
have to move on and face the truth, no matter
how painful and terrifying it may be. Remember,
though, God's Spirit dwells even here, in this
truth we so desperately wish we could avoid. As
we allow ourselves to become obedient to it, He
will purify our souls.

Clear my thoughts, Lord, so I can focus on You.
You know I don't want to accept this—but I
believe You can use even this to Your glory.

On the night before Your death, Jesus,
You prayed, "Let this cup pass from Me."
But in the end, You faced what lay before You.
You accepted the will of Your Father.
Give me strength, I pray, to do the same.

May the Trinity surround me now—
Father, Son, and Spirit. Encircle me,
I pray. Let me rest in Your reality.

I know that when I am weak, dear Christ, You
are still strong. Please renew my strength so that
I can face the facts. May Your Spirit sing songs of
hope within my soul. Awaken my heart, I pray,
so that I may accept the truth.

∽

I struggle to think clearly, God—so I depend
upon Your Spirit to illumine my mind. I am afraid
to face the darkness I sense gathering—so I look
to You for light. I don't want to accept this heavy
load—so I will give the burden to You. I wonder
if I am strong enough to take what lies ahead—
so I will rest for now in Your love and peace.

Bargaining with God

"Far be it from you to do such a thing! . . .
Will not the Judge of all the earth do right?"
GENESIS 18:25 NIV

∞

*P*sychologists recognize bargaining as another
way that we come to terms with a new and
frightening reality. When we pray, "Dear God,
if You'll only make this go away, I'll do this. . . ,"
we are being completely normal. And we're not
alone; even the great heroes of the Bible tried to
bargain with God.

Bargaining doesn't change reality. There's
nothing we can give to God that will make this
diagnosis go away. But God understands, and He
listens. We can be confident enough in His love
that we dare to say to Him whatever we feel. We
can even say, "God, don't do this! Why would You
let this happen? You know it's not right—so make
it go away!" We don't need to hesitate to come to
God with whatever is in our hearts.

How can I bear this, God? It's too much. I can't
do it. Please, God, *please* don't make me face this.

∞

Draw near to me, my loving Lord. Be with
me as I twist and turn, trying to escape this
diagnosis. Touch me. Hold me steady. Stand
between me and whatever lies ahead.

∞

Dear Jesus, I am throwing myself on You. I'm
pleading with You to send Your healing, as You
did with the crowds who followed You when
You walked this earth. I know I don't need to
persuade You to love me more than You already
do. I don't have to bribe You to have my best
interests always in mind. Your lovingkindness
is already with me, each step of the way.

Anger

Wake up, O Lord! Why do you sleep? Get up! Do not reject us forever. Why do you look the other way? Why do you ignore our suffering and oppression? . . . Rise up! Help us!
PSALM 44:23–24, 26 NLT

*M*odern Christianity doesn't talk much about being angry with God. We act as though our faith is supposed to be so great that it takes away our normal human reactions to terrible things like cancer. So when we find ourselves feeling angry with God because of cancer, we may think we need to pretend our anger isn't there. We may feel guilty voicing it.

But the psalmist had no problem venting all his rage into God's listening ears. And like him, we do not rage as if we have no promise of eternal justice. Our anger is contained by hope.

Lord Jesus, I have to confess that I feel angry with You. Why are You doing this to my family? Why won't You take this away from us? And Lord—thank You that You are big enough to handle my anger.

∞

God, I'm mad at You! Why did You let this happen? I know I should calm down and trust You—but my anger is just too big. I can't give You praise right now. I can't sing worship songs. The only thing I have to offer You is my anger. So here it is. I put it in Your hand.

∞

Loving Father, I feel as though being so angry with You has separated me from You. Remind me that that's a lie. Nothing can separate me from Your love—even my anger.

God, I know You are all-powerful. You are
strong enough to deal with my anger.
You can get me through this.

God, You are all-knowing. You love me
completely, and You know what's best for me.
You will never leave me, and You will meet
each and every need I have—even if You
do it in ways I don't expect.

When I hear the whisper that You are doing
this to punish me, because You are not really
a God of love after all, reassure me that this
whisper comes not from Your Spirit but
from Satan, the father of lies.

There is so much anger and confusion inside
of me, Jesus. I don't know what to think.
I can't focus on anything. Please heal me.
Strengthen me for whatever comes next.

∞

Jesus, as I say with You, "My God, my God,
why have You forsaken me?" (Matthew 27:46)—
may I also be able to pray, "Father, into Your
hands I commend my spirit" (Luke 23:46).

∞

In the end, God, You have not destined me for
anger but to obtain salvation through my Lord
Jesus Christ, who died for me so that whether I
am awake or asleep, alive in this world or in the
next world, I might live with Him. Therefore,
help me encourage my friends and family
who are also struggling now. May we build
up one another (1 Thessalonians 5:9–11).

Grief

*The LORD is near to the brokenhearted
and saves those who are crushed in spirit.*
PSALM 34:18 NASB

∞

*G*rief is yet another normal reaction to adjusting to a diagnosis of cancer, whether it's yours or a loved one's. Although a cancer diagnosis does not equal a death sentence, there are some things that *will* have to die, especially your plans for the immediate future. Letting go of professional plans, a longed-for family vacation, or some other short-term personal goal can seem not only disappointing but also devastating. We also feel sadness for the way in which cancer will affect everyone involved, especially children and young people. We are brokenhearted that they have to experience this now in their lives. Our spirits feel crushed.

Nothing anyone can say or do will force this sadness to disappear. Instead, we can simply rest, allowing ourselves to feel sad, knowing that God is near.

I'm waiting for You, Lord. I know You will lean down to me and hear my cry. You will draw me up out of the pit of destruction, this miry bog of grief and sadness where I'm stuck. You will set my feet on the rock, and You will make my steps steady. And then You will put a new song in my mouth, a song of praise to God. Many will see what You have done for me, and they, too, will put their trust in You (Psalm 40:1–3).

∞

Dear God, I feel as though cancer is a desert place, a barren and howling wasteland, where I'm lost, alone, heartbroken. Shield me, Lord. Care for me. Guard me as the apple of Your eye (Deuteronomy 32:10).

Heavenly Father, why is my soul so cast down?
Why do I feel such turmoil? Help me hope in
You. I know I will again praise You, for You are
my salvation and my God (Psalm 42:11).

I praise You, the Father of compassion and
the God of all comfort, who comforts me
now so that I will be able to comfort those
around me with the same comfort I receive
from God (2 Corinthians 1:3–4).

I am in distress; my eyes are sore with grief;
my soul and my body are exhausted.
My strength is gone, and my body has
let me down. Be gracious to me, O Lord.
Come and help me! (Psalm 31:9–10).

My comfort in this, God, is that Your
promises save me (Psalm 119:50).
Help me trust in them.

∞

Lord, You reached down from above. You took
and drew me up out of grief's deep waters. You
delivered me from my strong enemy, from this
sorrow that was too strong for me to overcome
on my own. When cancer threatened to knock
me off my feet, You held me steady. You brought
me forth into a large place, a place of freedom
and emotional health. You delivered me because
I delighted You (2 Samuel 22:17–20).

∞

My flesh and my heart may fail, Lord,
but You are the strength of my heart
and my portion forever (Psalm 73:26).

Why Me?

I pour out my complaints before
him and tell him all my troubles.
PSALM 142:2 NLT

∞

*D*on't feel guilty if you find yourself asking
God over and over why He has allowed this to
happen. That feeling is normal. It does not make
you less of a Christian. It won't even interfere
with your relationship with God, so long as you
share your feelings with Him. It may take a long
time before you get an answer. You may never
understand why this terrible disease has entered
your life.

Even Jesus experienced these same feelings.
On the cross, He asked His Father, "Why? Why
did You abandon me?" (Matthew 27:46). Like
Jesus, we, too, feel as though God has forgotten
about us.

But God answers our fears, saying to us,
"Can a mother forget her baby? Even if a mother
could forget her baby, I will never forget you!"
(Isaiah 49:15).

Why did this happen to me, Lord? Why me?
What did I ever do to deserve this? Remind me
that cancer is not a punishment for anything I
did. Use this disease to teach me compassion
for others. Be glorified even in cancer, I pray.

Help me, Jesus, to stop fretting. Instead, may
I turn my heart and mind to prayer, with
thanksgiving that You always hear me. I ask
that the peace of God, which surpasses all
understanding, will guard our hearts and our
minds in Christ Jesus. Help us stop focusing on
all that is wrong right now—and instead may
our thoughts and conversation dwell on all that
is honorable, whatever is pure, whatever is lovely,
whatever is admirable. Show us any excellence
in these happenings; reveal to us things that
are worthy of praise. Help us think about
those things (Philippians 4:6–8).

No matter how terrible things look right now,
I know that because You are my shepherd, Lord, I
have everything I need. Even though I'm walking
through the valley of the shadow of death, I
don't need to fear evil, for You are still with me.
Your rod and Your staff comfort me. You prepare
a table before me, right here in the presence of
cancer. You anoint my head with oil. My cup will
overflow with Your blessings (Psalm 23:1, 3–6).

God, I know You'll never desert me.
I know Your faithfulness will never end.

Acceptance

My health may fail, and my spirit may grow weak, but
God remains the strength of my heart; he is mine forever.
PSALM 73:26 NLT

∾

*A*ll of us will die. Most of us, however, spend
our lives hiding from that fact. We pretend that
it's not true. We act as though death is something
that happens only to other people, never to ourselves. But cancer forces us to face what has been
true all along: death is a reality with which we
must come to terms.

But with acceptance comes hope. We gain a
new understanding of what it means to have God
be the "strength of our heart." When He says,
"Forever," it's a promise. Nothing in this world
can make that promise, but God can.

I choose to bless Your name, Lord, even though I am facing cancer. I feel diminished by this disease—and yet I give You all that I have left to offer. Heal me, Lord, if it be Your will. Redeem my life from destruction. Crown me with Your lovingkindness and tender mercies (Psalm 103:1–4).

Teach us, God, to accept that cancer has entered our lives. I pray for healing (whether in this life or the next)—but in the meantime, give us strength to work with what we have right now. Help us focus on all that we still have, rather than on cancer. Make us useful to Your kingdom. Help our lives praise You.

God, I ask that You use cancer to teach me more about prayer. I know You do not always choose to answer my prayers as I want. I know that my perspectives are often too limited for me to even understand what I truly need most. And yet I believe You always hear my prayers. You never ignore me. My prayers always connect me to You—and they open up a space where You can work in me. Please work in me, Lord, in whatever way You choose.

∾

O my God, my life seems so dark. I don't know how to rise above this. Be my Sun, I pray. Rise over my life with healing in Your wings. Release me from cancer's chains that are holding me captive. Allow me to run free, like a calf that runs out of the barn when spring comes (Malachi 4:2).

Feelings of Doubt

Lord, I believe; help thou mine unbelief.
MARK 9:24 KJV

∞

*P*eter was walking along on the surface of the water, his eyes fixed on Jesus, doing just fine. Suddenly, he realized what he was doing. He looked at the waves beneath his feet, and he knew that what he was doing was *impossible*. Instantly, his feet sank into the water. He knew he was going to drown. But Jesus didn't let him. The Lord grabbed His good friend and saved him. And He will do the same for you.

Doubts recur, though. You don't ever seem to conquer them once and for all. And yet over and over, every time you're swamped with doubts and start to sink, Jesus will reach out His hand to you again. "Why do you doubt Me?" He asks each time. "Have I *ever* let you sink?"

I want to trust You, God. I want to give You all my fears. But no matter how many times I say the words, I can't follow through on them. I feel stuck. I'm helpless to change. Lord, I know You can do the impossible. Work a miracle in my heart, I pray.

I know, Jesus, that I am like a wave of the sea, driven and tossed by the wind (James 1:6). Doubts are like a storm all around me. But You say to me, "Why are you afraid, O you of little faith?" You have the power to quiet the storm (Matthew 8:26).

Dear God, when I read the Bible, I see that
I'm not the only one who had this problem.
Trust was just as hard for many of the great Bible
heroes. Jonah, for example, ended up inside a
whale because he couldn't trust Your commands.
Father, thank You that You never abandon me,
even when I fail to trust You. Even now, when
cancer is like a giant whale, swallowing my
entire life, You are here with me.

∞

God, You are the one who began a good
work in me (Philippians 1:6)—and I know
You will not walk away from me now.

Lord, I do trust You.
But help me trust You more.

∞

God, You know I still have doubts. But despite
my doubts, I affirm that neither life nor death,
neither angels nor any spiritual power, neither
height nor depth, nothing the future holds—in
fact, nothing whatsoever will ever be able to
separate me from Your love (Romans 8:38–39).

∞

I remain confident of this, Lord: I will see
Your goodness in the land of the living. I will
wait for You and take heart (Psalm 27:13–14).

Prayers for My Friends

And the LORD turned the captivity of Job,
when he prayed for his friends: also the LORD
gave Job twice as much as he had before.
JOB 42:10 KJV

∽

*C*ancer never affects just one person. When someone has cancer, everyone who loves that person will also be shaken. But by praying for one another, we free ourselves from the captivity of our own fears.

Friendship is what gives the body of Christ strength; we see God through our friends, and in turn, we show God to them. He speaks to us through their voices. He loves us through them. And in this dark time, we support each other in prayer. In the Lord, we give each other comfort and strength. We help each other face the pain and sorrow and fear. We set each other free to praise God.

Dearest Lord, heal this person I love who has cancer. You have promised to redeem our lives from destruction, and I pray now that You will crown this person with your lovingkindness and tender mercies (Psalm 103:4). Thank You that You always hear our prayers.

God, I know that all circumstances can lead us to You, even cancer. I pray that You would use this time of pain and illness to make our friendship stronger. May we give You glory.

I am so grateful, Lord, for the friends You've given me. I ask that You use our love for each other to bring health and healing to our hearts and bodies.

Dear Christ, thank You for Your body. Thank You that those who are strong in Your body help carry me when I am weak. When I am full of sadness and doubt, I rely on their faith. Give me strength one day to do the same for someone else.

∞

Thank You, God, for my friends. Thank You for all the ways I see Your face in them. I pray that they may see You in me as well, even in this dark time.

∞

As God's chosen people, holy and dearly loved, may my friends and I clothe ourselves with compassion, kindness, humility, gentleness, and patience. In this stressful time, help us bear with each other and forgive one another if we step on each other's toes. Help me forgive them for not being perfect, as You forgave me. May love surround us, binding us all together in perfect unity (Colossians 3:12).

Prayers for My Family

*If ye abide in me, and my words abide in you, ye shall
ask what ye will, and it shall be done unto you.*
JOHN 15:7 KJV

∾

*C*ancer adds to the stress of family life. Treatments, worries, physical illness, and heightened
emotions all contribute to an escalating sense of
tension that is hard on each member of the family.

Yet God can use this time to make our
family even stronger. When we find ways to meet
the challenges together, we draw closer to one
another. When we find ways to weather the crises
as they come along, we can thank God that He
has guided our family through the storm. Even in
the midst of cancer, He is building a strong and
beautiful foundation for our family's future.

My heavenly Father, I know that encouragement always goes two ways. When I encourage others, I, too, feel encouraged. Give me the strength to set aside my own fear and sadness so that I can encourage my family during this difficult time.

The members of our family are connected to each other, like parts of a body, a small version of Your Church, Lord. What hurts one of us hurts all of us. And what blesses one of us blesses all of us. In the midst of the hurt, Lord, send Your blessing.

Fill my loved ones from top to toe with Your healing Spirit, Jesus. May Your resurrection life bring healing and wellness into their being. May Your grace carry them through this hard time into a new season filled with hope and joy.

I pray for my loved ones, dear God, that they would be held at this time in Your loving arms. I know they're filled with fears. Comfort their hearts, I pray.

∞

Bless all of those with whom our family comes into contact during these days—doctors, nurses, aides, technicians—and make us a blessing to them. May they see Christ in us. And may we see Your face in theirs, sense Your touch in their hands, and trust them to bring Your healing power into our lives. Give us grateful hearts and gentle spirits. May those who talk with us sense that You live in us.

∞

Thank You, Lord, for my family, these people I love so much, who love me. I pray that You strengthen them and bless them. You know their needs, better than I do. May I not be so preoccupied with my own worries that I forget to show them how much I love them.

Prayers for My Spouse

Pray for each other so that you may be healed.
The prayer of a righteous person is powerful and effective.
JAMES 5:16 NIV

∞

*W*hen we're scared, in pain, and sad, sometimes we may forget that our spouses are also going through all of those same feelings. Worry can make us short-tempered with each other; it's always easy to vent all our negative feelings onto the person who loves us best. Here, too, we can turn to God in prayer. He is the only one who is big enough to carry all our anger and fear and sorrow. He understands our emotions, and no matter how unreasonable or emotional we are, His feelings won't be hurt. And He can then strengthen us so that we can love our spouses. Through His love, we can love them. And in His Spirit, we can lift them up in prayer.

Thank You, Lord, for my spouse's life. I am
so glad You brought this person into my life.
Without this partner in my life, I would not
be who I am today. We've been through hard
times together before—now, please help
us get through this as well.

∾

Loving Father, I know my spouse is scared,
just as I am. I pray that You would send Your
comfort. Encourage, uplift, and strengthen.
Give joy and a sense of peace, even in the
midst of all we're going through.

∾

Don't let cancer come between us, God.
Unite us in love. Make us stronger than we
have ever been. Help us help each other.

Just as You have encouraged me, Spirit of Love, help me encourage my spouse. You know I can't do it alone. Help me depend on Your grace.

Empower me, Lord, so that I can be strong enough to reach out in love to my spouse, giving my heart away anew, in this strange new reality where we find ourselves.

Give me patience and understanding, I ask, dear Jesus. Remind me that my spouse is also struggling. Help me have reasonable expectations of my spouse during this hard time. Instead of relying on them to meet all of my needs, let me rely only on You.

Prayers for My Children

Don't worry about anything; instead,
pray about everything. Tell God what you
need, and thank him for all he has done.
PHILIPPIANS 4:6 NLT

∞

*W*hen cancer touches our lives, our fears for
our children may be the hardest to bear. We feel
as though it's our job to protect them, to keep
them safe from fear—but cancer is an enemy
that's too big for us. We can't stand between it
and our children, sheltering them from its dark
shadow. We can't promise them that everything's
going to be all right, when we're not certain that
it will be. Our hearts break at the thought that
our children might have to face life without a
parent, when so many dangers already threaten
them in our uncertain world.

In the end, we must trust our children to
God's love, knowing that He loves them far more
than even we do.

Jesus, be with my children during this time.
Calm their fears. May they sense Your presence
with them and turn to You in a new way.

I trust my children to Your care, Father.
I know You will be with them even if I can't be.
May they know Your love is everlasting.

Being young is hard enough, Lord, without
all the extra stress of cancer. My children already
had so much to deal with between school and
activities, and now it seems nearly impossible
to give them the attention they need. Help
them not feel neglected, I pray. Give them new
maturity to understand. May they always
know how much I love them.

Lord, make my children strong in You and Your
mighty power. May they put on Your armor so
that they will be able to stand firm against all
strategies of the devil. Let them put on every
piece of Your armor so they will be able to resist
the enemy in the time of evil—and then after
the battle, they will still be standing firm. May
they put on the belt of truth and the body armor
of God's righteousness. Let their shoes be the
peace that comes from the Good News so that
they will be fully prepared. May they hold up
the shield of faith to stop the fiery arrows of the
devil, put on salvation as their helmet, and take
the sword of the Spirit, which is Your Word
(Ephesians 6:10–17).

∽

I know, God, that Your faithfulness will
reach through me to my children and their
children and *their* children (Psalm 100:5).

Prayers for My Medical Team

*I urge you, first of all, to pray for all people. Ask God to help
them; intercede on their behalf, and give thanks for them.*
1 TIMOTHY 2:1 NLT

∞

*C*ancer takes away our control. It asks that
we put our trust not only in God but also in
the doctors and other health-care professionals
who will be responsible for our treatment. As
adults who have grown accustomed to being
independent and making our own decisions,
it can be hard to yield to others' wisdom and
expertise. We may need to learn new lessons in
humility.

But God has put these specific people into
our lives—and we can thank Him for their care,
trusting that He will use them to be His hands
as they care for our bodies. He knows all things,
and He does all things well—and He can use this
time to teach us to become more like His Son.

Lord, I ask that You prepare all the doctors and
nurses so that they are able to focus. Enable them
to disregard any personal distractions so that
they will not overlook anything important.
I pray that each one is thinking clearly and able
to receive wisdom from You throughout all the
treatments. May every decision be correct
and every procedure be accurate.

∽

I pray for Your blessing, Jesus, on all the medical
equipment involved in treating this cancer
that has entered our lives. May it be working
perfectly. Bless the technicians and others who
are responsible for this equipment. Give them
eyes to see any problems, nimble hands,
and insight to understand.

Thank You, loving God, for these professionals
who will be fighting my cancer. May I not be
so self-centered, so preoccupied with my own
worries and pain, that I forget to see them
as human beings, individuals who are Your
children, with their own needs and concerns.
Help me sense when one of them is carrying an
extra burden. Make me quick to reach out with
kindness. May I be courteous and thoughtful,
even when I'm in pain. Make me a blessing to
them, as they are a blessing to me. May they
see Your Spirit alive in me.

∽

Lord, I know You are faithful. I ask that You
strengthen and protect all those on the medical
team (2 Thessalonians 3:3). Please fill me with
trust to listen and work with my doctors, to
believe that they have my best interest at heart,
and give me strength to not take my
frustrations out on them.

Physical Pain

Be very glad—for these trials make
you partners with Christ in his suffering.
1 PETER 4:13 NLT

∽

*J*esus experienced pain. He did not hold Himself separate from human experience, and He died on the cross in terrible agony. This means that He understands what we feel when we face the emotional and physical pains of cancer. We can turn to Him, knowing that even if no one else understands what we are going through, He truly understands.

Even more than that, through pain we can come to know Jesus better. As we allow His Spirit to work in us, we become partners with Him in a new way, sharing in His suffering on the cross.

Jesus, I don't know how to obey the apostle Paul
when he tells us to rejoice in our sufferings.
I will wait on You, though, believing that
somehow this suffering will produce endurance
. . .and endurance will produce strength of
character. . .and that hope will grow out of that,
a hope that will never be disappointed. Thank
You for pouring Your love into my heart
through the Holy Spirit (Romans 5:3–5).

∞

✓
Jesus, I feel as though I can't take this pain
anymore. It takes all my energy to handle it,
leaving me so little energy for anything else.
Please anoint me with Your strength. I surrender
this pain to You. Please carry it when I am too
weak—and if it be Your will, please take it from me.

God, this pain has taken control of my life. I feel weak and helpless. Discouragement, frustration, and resentment threaten to drown me. Lord, please show me the way forward. Allow me to find ways to control this pain. Teach me how to live with it. Transform it into something that leads me closer to You, I pray in Your name.

∽

Heavenly Father, please touch the area of discomfort and bring relief. Release the muscles that are tight, and bring Your restoration. May the pain retreat enough that sleep will be peaceful.

∽

Lord, this constant pain is a heavy burden. I cast it on You. Sustain me, I pray (Psalm 119:16).

Almighty God, You are the Creator, the master builder, the one who shaped our bodies before we were born. You breathe life into each cell and hold everything in place. Your Spirit lives in our earthly bodies. I ask now for Your Holy Spirit to move in this physical body. Bring relief from pain, I pray. Be Lord of this body and ease its discomforts.

You are our Savior, Jesus, who came to this earth to be with us in all our pain. Thank You that You are here now and that You are carrying this pain, too. Use this pain to draw me closer to You. May I learn to see pain as a way to share Your work on the cross.

Emotional and Spiritual Pain

*But the God of all grace, who hath called us unto his
eternal glory by Christ Jesus, after that ye have suffered a
while, make you perfect, stablish, strengthen, settle you.*
1 PETER 5:10 KJV

∞

Cancer is not only a disease of the body; it also
brings disease to our hearts and spirits. It fills us
with fear. It breaks our hearts. It robs us of our
normal daily joys. These emotions don't mean that
our faith has failed, though. The Gospels make
clear that Jesus suffered as much emotionally in
the garden, praying before His death, as He did
physically when He was actually hanging from
the cross. If Jesus could not escape this anguish,
then we should not expect to either. Instead of
fighting our emotions, trying to wrestle them into
submission, we can surrender them into God's
hands to do with them as He wills. Ultimately,
this pain will not make us weak—instead, it will
make us stronger!

Lord, You know all that I'm feeling right now. My heart hurts, and my spirit feels weak and wobbly. Remind me, Lord, that I am Your child, and even this emotional pain comes to me through Your loving hand. This hurts so much—but I believe that down the road a ways, I will reap a harvest of peace and righteousness from what I'm experiencing now (Hebrews 12:11).

I know, Jesus, that when You walked on the earth, You, too, felt the strain of emotional torment. Come beside me now, I ask, and lead me through this time when emotional strength is too weak to cope. Help me find peace and calm in Your presence.

Remind me, Holy Spirit, that this temporary
suffering is producing in me an everlasting weight
of glory, far beyond any comparison. Teach me
to focus less on feelings and more on that which
I can't perceive right now with my emotions.
Be more real to me, I pray, than any pain
(2 Corinthians 4:17–18).

∾

God, You promised to wipe every tear from
our eyes, because one day there will be no more
death or sorrow or crying or pain. All these
things will be gone forever (Revelation 21:4).
When my emotions overwhelm me,
remind me of that promise.

Isolation and Loneliness

*And I will pray the Father, and he shall give you another
Comforter, that he may abide with you for ever; even the
Spirit of truth. . .for he dwelleth with you, and shall be in you.*
JOHN 14:16–17 KJV

∾

*F*riends and family can offer precious support
and comfort during these dark days—but
ultimately each of us faces the pain of cancer
alone. No one else can stand in our shoes and
experience exactly what we are experiencing. No
matter how much we love each other, we can't
fully understand each other's feelings—and that
fact can seem like a wall that separates us from
the ones we love the most.

But in our loneliness, we are never truly alone.
The Comforter is with us. When no one else can
take away our loneliness, the Holy Spirit is con-
stantly present, speaking words of love that are for
our ears alone.

Lord, I feel so lonely. I don't want to burden the people I love with my feelings. I know they're dealing with their own emotions and reactions to this. Thank You that You're here with me. I'm counting on You in a way I never have before.

∞

What can separate me from Your love, Christ? Can troubles or pain or danger or illness? No, I know that in all these things You are with me. For I am sure that neither death nor life, nor angels nor rulers, nor things present nor things to come, nor powers, nor height nor depth, nor anything else in all creation will be able to separate me from the love of God in You, Christ Jesus my Lord (Romans 8:35–39).

Dear Jesus, I've grown used to clinging to other people for comfort. Help me avoid blaming them for not being able to help me now. Teach me to trust in You instead.

Jesus, when I read about Your death on the cross, I can tell You went through much of what I'm experiencing now. You felt lonely and forsaken. You wondered where God was. You felt death's pain and horror. And yet in the midst of all that, You still trusted Your Father. You put Your spirit in His hands. Help me follow Your example.

Lord, I'm realizing that when I reach the point where I have nothing left but You, I can finally realize that You alone are enough. You are the strength of my heart and my portion forever (Psalm 73:26).

Blessed be You, God, the Father of my Lord Jesus
Christ, for You are the Father of mercies and the
God of all comfort. You comfort me in all my
affliction, including this terrible loneliness. Use me
one day to comfort those who are going through
something similar. May I pass along the comfort
You give to me now (2 Corinthians 1:3–4).

∞

Even my closest friends don't understand
what I'm going through, Lord. But You do.
Your grace never fails me.

∞

Lord, I believe You are here with me, going
through this at my side. You will be with me;
You will not leave me or forsake me
(Deuteronomy 31:8).

Anxiety

Don't fret or worry. Instead of worrying, pray. Let petitions
and praises shape your worries into prayers, letting God
know your concerns. Before you know it, a sense of God's
wholeness, everything coming together for good, will come
and settle you down. It's wonderful what happens when
Christ displaces worry at the center of your life.
PHILIPPIANS 4:6–7 MSG

∞

*F*eeling anxiety when dealing with cancer is
another normal reaction, and we should never
think that anxiety means we have lost faith. In
fact, God can use anxiety to draw us closer to
Him, allowing us to recognize our need and limi-
tations, while turning to the One who is always
sufficient. God doesn't want us to let anxiety
destroy our lives, though, when there are still so
many ways He wants to bless us. He uses prayer
as a practical tool for helping us cope.

Why do I surrender my peace? Help me hope in You, knowing that soon I will be praising You for all You have done. You are the one who will make me smile again. You are my God (Psalm 43:5).

∞

Lord, help me stop feeling so anxious but instead, in every situation, with thanksgiving, remind me to turn to You in prayer. Thank You that Your peace, which goes beyond all understanding, will guard my heart and mind in Christ Jesus (Philippians 4:6–7).

∞

Because I dwell in the secret place of the Most High, Lord, I shall abide under the shadow of the Almighty. You are my refuge and my fortress, my God. In You I will trust. You have delivered me from all of life's snares and dangers. You have covered me with Your feathers, and under Your wings I take refuge. Your truth is my shield (Psalm 91:1–4).

I do not need to worry in the night, Lord, nor do I need to fret about dangers during the day. Neither sickness nor destruction is my concern. Even though people all around me are in trouble, I still don't need to worry, because You are my refuge. You—the Most High—are my dwelling place. You have given Your angels the job of looking after me. No matter what dangers I face, I am safe. Because of Your love, You will deliver me. You will set me in a high place. When I call on You, You answer me. If trouble comes, You will still be with me. You will deliver me and honor me. You will show me Your salvation all through my life. So why should I worry? (Psalm 91:5–16).

Lord, You are in complete control—and You are greater than any of my worries. I cannot change the future; I cannot change the circumstances of my life—so worrying is simply a waste of time and energy! Teach me that my energy could be better spent in prayer.

∞

Thank You, Father, for giving me the confidence that You are for me and with me. I know that life holds nothing that You can't overcome. No power is greater than You. I can rest in Your arms today, knowing that You have everything under control.

Help Me Relax, Lord!

"Oh, that I had the wings of a dove!
I would fly away and be at rest."
PSALM 55:6 NIV

∞

*N*o matter how much we know intellectually about God's strength and providence, and no matter how much faith we have spiritually, our bodies sometimes betray us. Our muscles are tense, preparing for a battle that we have no ability to fight. When we try to rest, our hearts pound and our stomachs hurt. Even though we turn our thoughts to prayer, our rebellious bodies still refuse to relax, and we lie there in the dark, hour after hour.

God is there, even in those moments. Take slow, deep breaths. Imagine yourself inhaling God's love, while you exhale all your tension. Don't try to think or pray beyond that. Simply breathe, one breath at a time.

You know how tense I feel, Lord, how unable to relax. After all, You made me, so You understand exactly how my body responds to this situation. Thank You that You never blame me for being human—but that You never leave me helpless, either. Your grace is always there, like a hand held out to me, waiting for me to reach out and grasp it.

Loving Jesus, I hear Your voice calling to me, "Come with Me into a quiet place and get some rest." So I am going away with You, into a place where You and I can be alone (Mark 6:31–32).

Thank You, Father, that You have promised
me peace. That in illness and even in death,
You will give me rest (Isaiah 57:2).

Teach me, Lord, to be still in Your presence.
Even in the midst of this terrible tension,
help me wait patiently for Your help (Psalm 37:7).

Jesus, I'm coming to You, burdened down
with stress. Give me Your rest. Show me
how to take Your yoke so that I may find
rest for my soul (Matthew 11:28–29).

Jehovah God, send Your presence with me.
Give me rest (Exodus 33:14).

God, because You are my shepherd, "you have
bedded me down in lush meadows, you find me
quiet pools to drink from. True to your word, you
let me catch my breath" (Psalm 23:1–3 MSG).

I am blessed, Lord, because I trust in You. My
confidence is in You alone. You make me like a
tree planted by the water, sending out my roots
by the stream. Despite the heat of the day, I don't
need to be afraid. You keep my leaves always
green. I don't need to get stressed about this time
of drought because You will make sure my life
still bears fruit (Jeremiah 17:7–8).

Praise in the Midst of the Worst

GOD is good, a hiding place in tough times.
He recognizes and welcomes anyone looking
for help, no matter how desperate the trouble.
NAHUM 1:7 MSG

∞

*C*oping with cancer is not easy. But as you get used to this new reality, you'll find that God is still bringing joy into your life. There will still be things that give you pleasure. Safe in God's hiding place, you can appreciate life's small pleasures: a beautiful sunrise, a child's smile, a friend's laughter. And no matter how desperate you feel at times, there are still so many reasons to praise God. The love others share with you takes on new meaning. You may even discover a new sense of purpose. God is waiting to bless you—so that you can praise Him even now.

I praise You, Lord, with all my soul. With all my inmost being, I praise Your holy name, I praise You, and I remember everything You have done for me. You forgave me, You redeemed me, You crowned me with love and compassion. You satisfy my desires with good things so that my youth is renewed like the eagle's (Psalm 103:1–5).

∞

I shout for joy to You, Lord. I worship You with gladness. I come before You with joyful songs. I know that You are God. You made me, and I am Yours. I am part of Your people, the sheep of Your pasture. I enter Your gates with thanksgiving and Your courts with praise. I give thanks to You and I praise Your name, even now. For You are good and Your love endures forever (Psalm 100).

Your love, Jesus, is as wide as the oceans, as deep as the sea, and as tall as the heavens. I praise You!

I called to You, Lord, out of my distress—and You answered me! When I was drowning, surrounded by an ocean of despair, with waves billowing over my head, I was sure that You were no longer paying attention to my life. I felt as though I was about to be destroyed. I was sure my life was over. But You brought me up from the pit of despair, Lord. You heard my prayer, even when I felt as though I was spiritually fainting. Lord, help me resist putting my trust in anything or anyone but You. When I do, I forsake my hope in Your steadfast love. My salvation comes from You! (Jonah 2:2–7).

You are the Lord of life! I hear You in the falling rain; I see You in the starry sky; I feel You in the warmth of the sun on my face. In each of these things, I give You praise.

Today, dear God, You blessed me. Let me take some time now to tell You how grateful I am. As I think back through my day, remind me of each joy, both big and small. Help me see all that is still good in my life.

Lord, You are my God. I will exalt You and praise Your name, for in perfect faithfulness You have done wonderful things, things You planned long ago (Isaiah 25:1).

When Others Don't Know What to Say

Bear with each other and forgive one another.
COLOSSIANS 3:13 NIV

∞

People often feel awkward in the presence of another's pain. What's more, the *C* word strikes fear into people's hearts. They don't know what to say. Sometimes they say silly things that may seem hurtful. Or they may be so worried that they will say the wrong thing that they say nothing at all—and that can hurt, too. We feel as though suddenly our very presence makes everyone feel uncomfortable.

Finding a cancer support group, where we can be with people who are going through the same thing we are, may be helpful. We can also learn to rely more on God for understanding than we may have in the past. And then we can forgive our well-meaning friends who don't know what to say.

God, how am I supposed to handle social situations now? People act so uncomfortable around me. They tiptoe around me awkwardly. Help me forgive them, Lord. I know I've probably acted the same way to others. Please send me someone who will let me cry, who will give me a hug, and who will sit and listen as I talk about my feelings. I know You understand— but please send me a human ear to also listen and understand!

∞

Dear Jesus, help me be more like You. You put up with so much from people who didn't understand You when You were on earth. May I follow Your example.

Lord, bless this person who hurt me with his words. Do good in his life. Bring good things to him. I ask that Your love would shine in his life.

∞

Help me forgive her, Jesus. Remind me how much You have forgiven me (Matthew 6:14).

∞

Help me, God, not to judge others for their words, since You have not judged me for all the times that I have spoken without understanding. Help me not condemn others, since You have not condemned me (Luke 6:37).

God, You know how angry I feel right now
with this person. You know how hurt I am.
Show me another perspective. Turn my
hurt feelings into Your love.

∾

Holy Spirit, fill me with Your love. Teach me not
to be so sensitive to slights and careless words.
Help me focus on others' needs, even when my
own seem so great. Teach me to love as You love.

∾

Make me tenderhearted, Lord, and forgiving
(Ephesians 4:32). Open my eyes to see
opportunities to be gentle, to be patient,
to be understanding of others.

When It's Time to Fight

God is strong, and he wants you strong. So take
everything the Master has set out for you, well-made
weapons of the best materials. And put them to use.
EPHESIANS 6:10–11 MSG

∞

*S*urrendering ourselves to God's will for our
lives doesn't mean we just lie back and give up on
life. We don't know what the future holds—but
we do know that God has a plan for our lives, and
He wants to bless us. With that perspective, we
can stand up and fight, refusing to let cancer have
the final word in our lives. We can take a stand to
hold on to love and hope and joy. No matter what
happens, cancer will not win—God will!

God, help me put on Your entire armor,
that I may be able to withstand everything
cancer throws at me—and having done all,
to stand firm (Ephesians 6:13).

Thank You, Lord, that I do not have to fight
this battle. I'm taking my position, I'm standing firm, and I'm waiting to see the deliverance
You will give me. Help me resist being afraid
or discouraged. I'm going to go out there
and face cancer—and I know You will be
with me (2 Chronicles 20:17).

When the storm has swept by, I will still be
standing firm—forever (Proverbs 10:25).

Lord, don't let anything move me. Help me always give myself fully to Your work, knowing that nothing I do for You is ever in vain (1 Corinthians 15:58).

Take away my fear, Lord, and help me stand firm, waiting to see the deliverance You will bring me. Cancer better run and hide! You are fighting for me. All I need to do is be still and rely on You (Exodus 14:13–14).

Whatever happens, heavenly Father, help me conduct myself in a manner worthy of the Gospel of Christ. I want to stand firm in Your Spirit, spreading the Good News even now (Philippians 1:27).

Jesus, You promised that if I stand firm, I'll win life. So I'm taking my stand! (Luke 21:19).

∽

God, show me how to put on Your full armor so that when cancer does its worse, I'll be able to stand my ground—and after I've done everything I know how to do, to just keep on standing. Give me a firm stance. Buckle Your truth around my waist. Put Your breastplate of righteousness in place, and slide Gospel shoes onto my feet so that I'll always be ready to carry Your peace out into the world (Ephesians 6:13–15). You and I together, Lord—we're not going to let cancer have the last word!

∽

It is for freedom that You set me free, Christ, so help me stand firm. Don't let me allow myself be burdened again by a yoke of slavery to fear (Galatians 5:1).

Feeling Bad Isn't Giving Up

When he falls, he will not be hurled headlong,
because the LORD is the One who holds his hand.
PSALM 37:24 NASB

∞

*O*ne day we decide to stand up and fight—and
the next day we're too sick to move. When that
happens, discouragement can knock us down
even lower. But feeling sick, feeling sad, feeling
weak, and feeling scared are all normal human
emotions. No one is a superhero, and cancer is a
formidable enemy. Ask soldiers who have gone
into battle, and you'll find that most, if not all,
of them were afraid. They may have felt sick and
weak, but they stood up and fought anyway. They
did what they had to. Feeling bad doesn't mean
we've given up!

Plead my cause, Lord, against cancer. Fight against it on my behalf. Take up Your shield and armor when I'm too weak to lift them. Arise and come to my aid. Brandish Your spear and javelin against cancer. Let me hear Your voice saying, "I am your salvation." May all the cancer cells be destroyed and put to shame; may they give up and turn back. May they be like chaff before the wind, with the angel of the Lord driving them away! Then my soul will rejoice in You and delight in Your salvation. My whole being will exclaim, "Who is like You, Lord? You rescue the weak when cancer is too strong for them, the poor and needy from the cancer cells that would rob them of life (Psalm 35:1–6, 9–10).

When my prayers returned to me unanswered,
I was depressed. I bowed my head and cried,
as though I had lost my last friend. When I
stumbled, my enemy seemed to gather against
me even stronger. Lord, You see what's going
on—don't keep silent! Don't be far from me,
Lord. Awake, and rise to my defense! Stand
up for me, my God and Lord. Vindicate me in
Your righteousness, Lord my God; do not let
cancer gloat over me. Do not let cancer think
it has swallowed me up. Put each cancer cell
to shame! May those who are praying for me
shout with joy and gladness. May they say, "The
Lord be exalted, who delights in the well-being
of His servant." My tongue will proclaim Your
righteousness and Your praises all day long
(Psalm 35:13–15, 22–28).

Surgery

"The LORD himself goes before you and will be with you; he will never leave you nor forsake you. Do not be afraid; do not be discouraged."

DEUTERONOMY 31:8 NIV

∞

*H*ave you ever done that exercise in trust where you fall backward into another person's arms? It's hard to let yourself drop, trusting that the other person will catch you. In the same way, as we go into surgery, surrendering to the anesthesiologist, our hearts are filled with fear. We go under, uncertain what we will find when we wake up. It seems a little like death, a venture into a dark and unknown place. We are forced to trust the medical team's skill.

But at the same time, we can also commit ourselves to God's unfailing love, letting ourselves drop into His hands. While we are unconscious, He will be awake. His hands are sure, and He will hold us safe.

As I go into the operating room, I will rest in Your promises, loving Lord. I will lean back into Your love for me, sinking into Your peace as the surgeons work. Remind me that You are there with them, in them. Your Spirit is working in their hands to bring restoration to my body. I lie down holding Your hand that has never let me go, all the days of my life, believing that You will lead me into new seasons filled with hope. I know that when I am most vulnerable, You will be with me, that Your love will hold me safe.

∾

Today, as I go into surgery, give me the courage, Jesus, to say the words You spoke on the cross: "Into your hands I commit my spirit" (Luke 23:46 NIV).

Jesus, my best friend, You know how scared I am as I face this surgery. What if something goes wrong? What if there are complications? Will I ever feel like myself again? How much pain will I have to face during the recovery process? In the midst of all these fears, Lord, I cling to You. Yes, I'm terrified—but I nevertheless trust You.

∞

Lord, You are the author of life, the Great Healer. You know all that is wrong inside my body. Please be with me during this surgery. Breathe Your peace into my heart. Be with my family as they wait. Assure them that You are in control.

∞

Jesus, may the doctors and nurses who care for me today, before and after the surgery, sense Your presence in me. Bless them through me, I pray.

Lord, You told us not to worry about tomorrow. Thank You that You pour out Your Spirit upon us anew each day, even on days like this one. Thank You that Your grace is sufficient for us in each moment that we live, even this moment as we face surgery (2 Corinthians 12:9).

∞

Lord, I place my loved one in Your hands today. Guide the medical professionals who will do the surgery. Give them skill and wisdom, sure hands and alert minds. Use them to restore health so that You may be glorified.

God of power and might, guide the surgeon's hands, I pray. May our loved one's body respond quickly to this treatment. May this person we love be healed to serve You anew.

As I lie on the operating table, may I know Your peace in my heart, Jesus, a peace that surpasses all understanding, that will guard my heart and mind (Philippians 4:7).

Holy Spirit, as I undergo this surgery, come and be present with me, watching and waiting, ready to help and guard me every moment during this procedure. Hold me in Your love, and protect me from all harm.

Will I Ever Feel Normal Again?

"I am with you, and I will protect you wherever you go. One day I will bring you back to this land. I will not leave you until I have finished giving you everything I have promised you."

GENESIS 28:15 NLT

∞

*B*efore the surgery, we may have felt as though once it was over, life could begin to get back to normal. Instead, we are faced with new pains and new weakness. "Normal life" seems like a distant memory. Our old competent selves seem as though they've disappeared forever.

But in this time of weakness and pain, God's promises still hold true. He has a future planned for us, a future that is full of blessing, and He has work He needs us to do for His kingdom. For now, though, He wants us to wait for His timing. We have important lessons to learn during this time when normal life has retreated into the distance, lessons that will make us strong for the work ahead.

I hate feeling like this, Lord. I don't like not feeling like my old self. I don't like being an invalid. I want to get up and get my old life back. I'm so frustrated, so discouraged. Lord, I need You.

∽∞

Forgive me, Jesus, for wanting to be able to do things for myself again. Forgive me for wanting to be in control. Forgive me for complaining and grumbling. Help me avoid doubting Your love. Help me to trust You.

∽∞

When I question what the future will hold, God, help me trust You. Use this time to Your glory.

I bow my knees before You, Father, that according to the riches of Your glory You will grant me to be strengthened with power through Your Spirit in my inner being so that Christ may dwell in my heart through faith. Root me and ground me in love so that I may have strength to comprehend with all the saints what is the breadth and length and height and depth of Your love. Use this time of pain and weakness to help me understand the love of Christ that surpasses knowledge, that I may be filled with all Your fullness of God. I know You are able to do far more abundantly than all that I ask or think, according to the power at work within me. To You, Lord, be glory in the Church and in Christ Jesus throughout all generations, forever and ever! (Ephesians 3:14–21).

When All Seems Hopeless

Blessed be the Lord—day after day he carries us along. He's
our Savior, our God, oh yes! He's God-for-us, he's God-
who-saves-us. Lord GOD knows all death's ins and outs.
PSALM 68:19–20 MSG

∞

$\mathcal{W}$e tend to think of hope as a cheery, opti-
mistic outlook on life. But the biblical concept of
hope is far greater and deeper. It is a confidence
and expectation in what God will do in the future,
an understanding that the same God who was with
us yesterday will be with us tomorrow. Cancer can
rob us of this confidence. It can convince us that
there is no hope. We feel as though the future is
empty and barren.

But hopelessness is always a lie, for our God
has big plans for us! No matter where the road
ahead takes us, it always leads us into His presence.

When I feel hopeless, Jesus, remind me that You love me just as much as Your Father loves You. You—the Son of God, the Word that existed from before the beginning of the world—love me, infinitely, unconditionally, with all Your heart! May I take hope in Your love.

Remind me, loving Lord, that the world I see with my physical eyes is only a piece of reality, a glimpse into an enormous and mysterious universe. Even if I can't see what's going on, You are doing amazing, mysterious, beautiful things!

Praise be to You, the God and Father of my Lord Jesus Christ! In Your great mercy You have given me new birth into a living hope through the resurrection of Jesus Christ from the dead. Through Jesus, I have an inheritance that can never perish, spoil, or fade. This inheritance is kept in heaven for me, and in the meantime, through faith I am shielded by God's power until the coming of the salvation You will eventually reveal to me. Remind me that even though I have to suffer grief and trials for a little while now, I can still rejoice in You, my God of living hope (1 Peter 1:3–6).

When I can't sense Your presence with me, God, give me grace to believe that I will one day soon experience Your joy again.

I'm groaning in my heart, Lord, moaning
and crying out for You. My body needs Your
salvation. This is the hope that saves me. And
I know that if I didn't have to wait for Your
healing, I wouldn't need to hope. Who hopes for
what they already have? So I hope for what I do
not yet have, waiting, trying to be patient, while
Your Spirit helps my weakness. I don't even
know how to pray; I don't know what I should
ask You to do—but Your Spirit intercedes for
me. And I know that in all things You work for
my good, working to shape me into the image
of Your Son (Romans 8:24–29).

When I Feel Helpless

I am well content with weaknesses. . .
for when I am weak, then I am strong.
2 CORINTHIANS 12:10 NASB

∽

e've all heard the expression "God helps those who help themselves." And while there's a certain truth to the saying—God doesn't want us to sit there expecting a miracle when He's already put the means to accomplish something into our hands—the opposite is also true: God helps those who are helpless. Look at the tax collector in the Gospel who didn't even try to prove his worth but instead just stood off at a distance and threw himself on God's mercy (Luke 18:13). Jesus said, "Blessed are the poor in spirit, for theirs is the kingdom of heaven" (Matthew 5:3 NIV). When we are helpless, when we give up our dependence on our own strength, then God can begin to act in our lives.

Lord, You promise to give me all that I need.
I depend on You for my help.

Jesus, I can't control my life anymore. I don't
know where to turn. I give up. Please, take over.

I know You have the strength I need,
heavenly Father. Give me a new perspective,
I pray. Instead of worrying about my own
weakness, help me glory in Your power.

Since I am surrounded by such a huge crowd of witnesses to the life of faith, help me, dear Jesus, to strip off every weight that slows me down, especially the sin that so easily trips me up. Help me run with endurance the race You have set before me, even though it leads me on this track through cancer. I know that keeping my eyes on You, the champion who initiates and perfects my faith, is the only way I'll have strength to do this. Because of the joy awaiting You, You endured the cross, disregarding its shame—so if You did that, I know You can give me the strength I need to put up with cancer! When I feel like giving up, remind me of all You endured for me (Hebrews 12:1–3).

I need You, God. I can't handle life on my own.

Lord, You know the hopes of the helpless.
Surely You will hear my cries and
comfort me (Psalm 10:17).

Thank You, God, for pouring out Your love
into my heart through the Holy Spirit, whom
You have given to me. For at just the right time,
when I was completely helpless, Christ came
and gave Himself for me (Romans 5:5–6).

Recovery from Surgery

We are troubled on every side, yet not distressed; we are perplexed, but not in despair; persecuted, but not forsaken; cast down, but not destroyed; always bearing about in the body the dying of the Lord Jesus, that the life also of Jesus might be made manifest in our body.
2 CORINTHIANS 4:8–10 KJV

∞

Recovery is a long, slow process. Most people realize that their bodies will need time to recover after undergoing a surgical procedure, but we may forget that our hearts and minds also need time to heal. At the same time that we work to build our bodies' strength back to what it was before, we need to do everything we can to also restore ourselves spiritually and emotionally. A healthy diet is important, as well as exercise and plenty of rest—both physically and spiritually. More than ever, we need to be sure we are consuming that which is truly nourishing rather than "junk food." By spending extra time in prayer and scripture reading, we can speed our spiritual and emotional recovery—and that will be good for our bodies' healing as well.

Touch me, heal me, restore me, redeem me.
Come and be Lord in this situation. I open
my heart and mind and body to Your power.

Strengthen me, empower me, use me. You were
with me each step of the way, Jesus,
and I know You will not leave me now. You
watched over me through the surgery. Your angels
stood guard around me. Now I pray for rest and
peace. May I dwell in Your love and truth.

I praise You, Lord, with all my soul. I remember all
You have done for me. You not only have forgiven
all my sins, but You also heal me in every way. You
have redeemed me, and now You crown me with
Your love and compassion (Psalm 103:2–4).

Wrap me in Your love, God. Hide me deep within Your wings. Breathe Your Spirit's healing into me, body and soul. Restore me so that I may serve You.

Thank You, loving Lord, for the doctors and nurses who cared for me. Continue to bless the work of their hands.

I will keep my eyes on You, Lord, and use this time to draw still closer to You. I give You all that I am, and I rest in Your peace. I hold tightly to Your promises.

Lord, heal me, and I will be completely well. Rescue me, and I will be perfectly safe. You are the one I praise! (Jeremiah 17:14).

Chemotherapy

For I consider that the sufferings of this present
time are not worthy to be compared with
the glory that is to be revealed to us.
ROMANS 8:18 NASB

∞

Chemotherapy demands our physical atten-
tion, and it's hard to feel as though this is a spiritual experience. Our bodies' discomfort may make
us feel as though we are far from God. But that's
only an illusion! God is as close to us as ever, and
He longs to be with us, no matter what we're
going through. Scientific research has even found
that those who pray throughout their treatments,
actively living out a life of faith while undergoing
this process, actually respond more quickly and
fully. God is the Lord of cancer cells as well!

Lord, the world of science tells me that only what can be seen and measured is truly real. But my heart knows differently. Every day, I depend on You. I may not be able to see You with my physical eyes, but You are the one who gives me grace to live through these days.

∞

As I go through these uncomfortable treatments, heavenly Father, I lift up all the other patients who are also undergoing this. Please be with them, as I know You have been with me. Give them comfort and peace during this battle. Bring them healing. And be with all our families, too, as they travel with us on this long, hard journey.

Radiation

Have compassion on me, LORD, for I am weak.
Heal me, LORD, for my bones are in agony.
PSALM 6:2 NLT

∞

Radiation treatments wear us down, mentally, physically, spiritually. We may feel as though we've finally reached the end of our strength. After all we've already gone through, how can God expect us to endure any more?

And yet others before us have found God even in the midst of terrible discomforts. Aleksandr Solzhenitsyn, the Russian author who spent ten years in a Soviet work camp, wrote, "I nourished my soul there, and I say without hesitation: 'Bless you, prison, for having been in my life.'" The prophet Isaiah also learned to see a purpose in the pain he had endured: "Surely it was for my benefit that I suffered such anguish" (38:17 NIV).

When we reach the end of our rope—we'll find God already there, His hand held out to catch us.

When I get to the end of my rope, dear Lord, remind me to take Your hand. Thank You that You have all the strength I'll ever need. Teach me to rely on You instead of on my own strength. I know that when I do, You'll help me to endure. You'll get me through this.

Today I ask by faith that You bring healing from these treatments. You taught us, Lord Jesus, that faith as small as a mustard seed can grow into a tree. Today all I have left is a little seed of faith—but I give it to You. I place it in the ground of Your Word, and I water it with Your truth. I know the warmth of Your love will make it grow.

As I lie here receiving this radiation into my body,
I choose, O God, to see this as a gift, a dose
of Your healing energy. As I receive it, I imagine
Your light routing the enemy from my body.
I picture Your energy bringing me physical and
spiritual well-being. My body, mind, and spirit
gratefully receive this gift. I surrender to
Your healing of my total being.

Great Physician, I ask that You destroy all
the cancer cells. May Your healing virtue flow
through every cell. Bring health and restoration.

In the midst of this, Lord, feed me with
Your nourishment. Renew me. Help me
fly like an eagle! (Psalm 103:5).

Dealing with the Side Effects

Therefore we do not lose heart.
Though outwardly we are wasting away,
yet inwardly we are being renewed day by day.
2 CORINTHIANS 4:16 NIV

∞

*S*ometimes the treatment can seem as bad as the disease. We may have thought we knew what to expect, but the reality can be worse than we imagined. Nausea robs joy from our days. Hair loss can make us feel as though we have changed into someone we don't even recognize when we look in the mirror. "Chemo brain" can make it difficult for us to concentrate on prayer—or anything else!

During times like these, just enduring is enough. This period in our lives will not last forever. We tell ourselves we can hold on one more minute, one more hour, one more day—and we do. We let God take care of our inward renewal, day by day. Our job is simply to hold on.

Lord, You are the fountain of life. I ask for
Your life-giving water to pour down on me.

Jesus, if even the wind and the sea obeyed You,
I know You can handle my rebellious body.
Nothing is beyond Your power.

Abba, loving Father, I know You understand
what I'm going through. I cling to You.

Help me, God, to not be afraid or dismayed as
I experience these side effects. You are my God,
and I know You will strengthen me and help me.
I ask You to uphold me with the right hand
of Your righteousness (Isaiah 41:10).

Dear God, I dwell in Your house. Help me find peace and rest in Your presence.

Thank You, Jesus, that You were willing to go through such pain and suffering on my behalf. Please use the discomfort and pain of this time to draw me closer to You.

I believe in the power of Your name, Lord Jesus. I place my trust in You, no matter what. I wait for Your healing. You are my hope.

My comfort in my suffering is this: Your promise preserves my life (Psalm 119:50).

Physical Weakness

But those who trust in the LORD will find new strength.
They will soar high on wings like eagles. They will run
and not grow weary. They will walk and not faint.
ISAIAH 40:31 NLT

∞

*P*hysical weakness is hard to bear. We want to
be *better*. We want our old lives back. We want
our bodies to be the way they used to be, capable
of doing all that they once did. We have days
when we ask ourselves, "How much further can
I go? How much longer can I keep on like this?"
Days like that, we long to give up. We feel too
weak to keep going.

All we can do now is turn again to the Lord,
trusting that He will give us new strength—
not only to walk through our days without
fainting but also to soar on eagle wings. When
we acknowledge our own weakness, that's the
moment when the Holy Spirit can begin to work
in our lives in new ways.

Lord, You know how weak I am. But I can do all things through You because You give me strength (Philippians 4:13).

Heavenly Father, make me strong in You. May my strength come from Your might (Ephesians 6:10).

Jesus, I'm so weak, so exhausted. I'm not sure I can go on. I just want to give up. So take over. Do for me what I'm too weak to do for myself.

God, the Bible says that a merry heart will do me good (Proverbs 17:22). Give me reasons to laugh today, I pray.

Jesus, You know that my spirit is willing, but my flesh is weak. Remind me to keep watching and praying (Matthew 26:41).

∞

If by faith Sarah was able to have a baby, even when she was old (Hebrews 11:11), Lord God, I believe You can also work miracles in my body. Put new life in me that I may serve You once again.

∞

Spirit of Truth, I know You satisfy those who are weary and refresh everyone who is weak (Jeremiah 31:25). Come to my aid now, I pray.

Emotional and Spiritual Weakness

*"My grace is all you need.
My power works best in weakness."*
2 CORINTHIANS 12:9 NLT

∞

When we feel as though we're too weak to accomplish anything, we often feel blue and depressed. Our physical weakness makes us feel equally weak emotionally and spiritually. Our self-concepts suffer. We measure ourselves against what we used to be, and we come up lacking.

But it doesn't have to be that way. When we stop focusing on our own lack and instead turn our eyes to God, He has a chance to reveal His mighty power. His grace will be revealed in our lives. In fact, we may experience His grace and strength in new ways, more powerfully than ever before.

I am so weak, God. But You promised me that Your power is made perfect in weakness, that Your grace is all I need. Here, God. I put my weakness in Your hands. Use it however You want. May Your grace fill my life.

∞

I'm tired of being sick, Lord. The challenge is too big for me. My self-confidence fails. I can't help but compare how big the challenge is to my meager abilities for confronting it. My faith wavers. Help me.

∞

Jesus, I believe I can do all things—because You make me strong (Philippians 4:13).

I know, dear Jesus, that when I admit how weak
I truly am, then You have the chance to reveal
Your strength. The challenge that lies ahead
shrinks when I compare it to Your immensity.
Keep me focused on You and Your power.

∞

Therefore, Christ, I'll be content with weakness
and distresses and difficulties, for Your sake, for I
know that when I am weak, then I am strong—
because of You (2 Corinthians 12:10).

∞

Father, You give strength to the weary, and
when we lack strength, You give us power.
Though young people with their strong, healthy
bodies get tired and stumble, I will have new
strength to keep going—because I am waiting
only for You (Isaiah 40:29–31).

Crying Out to God

*In my distress I called upon the Lord,
and cried unto my God: he heard my voice. . .
and my cry came before him, even into his ears.*
PSALM 18:6 KJV

∞

*C*rying out to God is an act of desperation. In the Bible, whenever we read that someone cries out to God, it is also a fervent expression of faith and trust. Just as a baby cries, knowing that the sound of her voice will bring her mother to her, crying out to God expresses our confidence in His love, as well as His power to act on our behalf. It expresses our humility, surrender, and faith.

And God hears our cries. The Bible is filled with examples of times when God answered the cries of His people. Like a loving mother, He comes to us when we cry for Him. He will not leave us to cry alone.

Without You, Lord, I can do nothing
(John 15:5). Help me!

In my distress I called upon You, Lord,
and I cried out to You—and You heard
my voice out of Your temple. My cry
reached Your ears (Psalm 18:6).

Jesus, Son of David,
have mercy on me! (Mark 10:47).

Fulfill the desire of my heart, dear God.
Hear my cry and save me! (Psalm 145:19).

Lord of heaven, I need Your help. I ask for restoration of body and mind. I ask for increased faith and new strength. You are my Lord, my Savior—and You are my healer and my friend. I'm counting on You.

It is because of Your mercy, Lord, that I am not consumed, because Your compassion never fails. Your love for me is new every morning. Great is Your faithfulness (Lamentations 3:22–23).

When I cry out to You, loving God, my enemies turn back—for You are on my side (Psalm 56:9).

Dear God, I feel so tired and sad. My heart is bruised. I feel abandoned, beaten. I've lost my sense of hope. And so I come to You. All I have left to give You are broken pieces. Put me back together again, I pray. Make me new.

∞

Help! Sometimes that's the only word I can think of to pray. Thank You, heavenly Father, that I don't need to speak complicated and eloquent prayers. You always hear my cry— even when all I can say is a single word.

∞

I'm lost! Please come and find me, Lord. I need You! Bring me back into Your presence. Show me the way.

Shame

For the Lord GOD will help me; therefore shall I
not be confounded: therefore have I set my face like
a flint, and I know that I shall not be ashamed.
ISAIAH 50:7 KJV

∾

*S*hame is that terrible, secret feeling that
something is wrong with us. Cancer can make us
feel like that, as though we will never be normal
again, that we are irreparably damaged. Our sense
of shame can attach to old feelings of inadequacy
that we've been carrying since childhood,
convincing us that we are somehow defective as
human beings.

When Jesus faced His death on the cross,
the Bible says He "endured the cross, scorning its
shame" (Hebrews 12:2 NIV). Jesus went through
the suffering—but He rejected the shame. He
was being treated as a person with no value—but
Jesus refused to accept it. Shame is always a lie.
We are not inadequate or defective—and we are
loved and cherished by God.

Jesus, when You encountered disease, You saw it as simply an opportunity for Your Father to display His power through You. You knew that these physical conditions had nothing to do with sin, nor did they mean that the individual was any less worthy of respect and honor. May I have that same confidence now.

∾

Holy Spirit, help me let go of this sense of shame. It keeps me focused on how bad I feel about myself, and that makes me less aware of You, less sensitive to others' needs. Shame immobilizes me. It isolates me. Break down the walls of shame that enclose me, I pray. Set me free.

Thank You, Christ Jesus, that there is no condemnation for those who are in You. I know that the law of the Spirit of life has set me free in You from the law of sin and death, for God has done what nothing else could do for me. By sending You to earth wearing the same sort of body that I do, God destroyed everything that separates me from Him. His righteousness is fulfilled in me, and now I can walk in the Spirit rather than in my own strength. I'm going to stop focusing on physical problems and set my mind on the things of Your Spirit. Help me live by Your power (Romans 8:1–3).

God, when people feel so uncomfortable with my disease, I start to feel ashamed of it, as though it's a dirty secret I shouldn't talk about. Give me courage to hold my head high, knowing that You have been with me through this long journey. I have nothing to be ashamed of.

∽∞

I can't help but wonder sometimes, Lord— did I do something bad that brought this cancer on me? Did I expose myself to something physically that I should not have? Did my negative thoughts make cancer cells grow inside my body? Were You punishing me for something I did wrong? Lord, release me from these thoughts. No matter how many times they pop into my mind, remind me over and over that these thoughts are lies. I am perfect in Your sight.

Asking Others for Help

*"You will surely wear out. . .for the task
is too heavy for you; you cannot do it alone."*
EXODUS 18:18 NASB

∞

*S*ometimes it's hard to admit that we need
help. We don't want to be a burden on others.
We don't want people to think we're weak. And
we don't like to feel as though we can't still be
independent, in control of our own lives.

But the Bible talks about the body of Christ
because God knows that we need each other
in order to thrive and serve Him. None of us
could make it in life without the help of others.
Sometimes we may need more help, sometimes
less. One day it will be our turn to help others.
For now, we need to have the humility and grace
to accept the help we need.

Is it pride that's standing in my way of asking others for help, Lord? If that's the case, then help me find the will to be humble.

Jesus, help me resist thinking I'm better than I really am, that I'm too good to ask for help. Enable me to be honest in my self-evaluation. I know that You have made us to be many parts of Your one body and that we all belong to each other. In Your grace, You have given us each gifts to use differently for each other's benefit (Romans 12:3–6). Thank You for giving me Your help through the hands of others. May I have the grace to accept the help I need.

Your Word tells us that we all have different kinds of gifts to offer—but all of them serve You. You work in different ways through each of us, but You are always the same God. You hand out these gifts to each of us and decide whom You need to do each task. Just as my physical body has many parts, so does Your spiritual body, all of us baptized into this body by one Spirit that we all share. I know it wouldn't make sense for my foot to say, "I'm not part of the body because I'm not a hand"— and it doesn't make sense for me to say, "Because I need help right now, I'm not worth as much as others are" (1 Corinthians 14:4–5, 12–16).

Keep reminding me, heavenly Father, that if my ear said, "I'm not as good because I'm not an eye," that would be silly—and I'm also being silly when I say to myself, "I'm not as good as my friend who is so strong and capable." You have put me just where You want me in Your body. Just as my eye can't say to my hand, "I don't need you," I can't say to my friends and family, "I don't need your help" (1 Corinthians 12:17–21).

∞

Dear Lord, You tell me that even when I am weak and in need of others' help, I still serve You. Some parts of the body that seem weakest and least important are actually the most necessary. I thank You for Your honor and care, Lord. Thank You that You made us to serve You by caring for each other (1 Corinthians 12:22–23).

Taking Care of Myself

Seize life! Eat bread with gusto, drink wine with a robust
heart. Oh yes—God takes pleasure in your pleasure! Dress
festively every morning. Don't skimp on colors and scarves.
Relish life with the spouse you love each and every day
of your precarious life. Each day is God's gift.
ECCLESIASTES 9:7–9 MSG

∽

*A*s we pray for healing and strength, we
need to do our part as well. We need to eat foods
that will speed our healing—healthy fruits and
vegetables, whole grains, lean protein—and make
time for prayer and quiet that will help to heal
our souls. Like a loving mother, God delights
in nourishing His children, but He won't force-
feed us! We also need rest, both physically and
spiritually, so we need to remember to not push
ourselves too hard. But even more than life's
basics, as we regain our strength, we need to begin
to take pleasure in life once more. Put on our best
clothes! Enjoy our spouses! Accept each day as a
precious gift from God.

Remind me, heavenly Father, to take care of myself. I know others need me—You need me—and *I* need me (as funny as that sounds). Help me take time to eat healthy meals. Give me the gift of sleep and relaxation. Remind me to exercise, even if it's just going for a walk.
Show me life's small pleasures.

"At day's end I'm ready for sound sleep, for you, God, have put my life back together" (Psalm 4:8 MSG). I can sleep in peace, knowing that meanwhile You will continue to work, healing everything in my mind, body, and soul that still needs Your touch. You renew me in my sleep.

Lord, after all that my body has been through,
it deserves my care and attention. I want to
dress attractively—and feel good about myself.
I want to enjoy touching and being touched.
I want to be alive!

∞

I praise You, Lord, for all that You have given
me—for all the things I used to take for granted.
Thank You not only for food to eat but also for
an appetite. Thank You not only for opportunities
to exercise but also for the strength to be able
to move around again. Thank You not only for
times of rest but also for the ability to fall asleep
without pain. You are so good to me!

Remind me, Father, that I am Your temple. Your
Spirit dwells in me. That makes me holy—so I
need to take care of myself (1 Corinthians 3:16).
I need to make sure Your temple is well cared for,
swept out, the windows open, the rooms all
filled with flowers and song and joy.

Let me not give myself to anything that draws
me away from You, Lord, for I know those things
will not lead to my health and healing. Instead,
I give myself to You. You have brought me back
to life. Please use me as an instrument for Your
righteousness (Romans 6:13)—and I know that
will be the best way I can speed my recovery.

Loving My Body

What? know ye not that your body is the temple
of the Holy Ghost which is in you, which ye have
of God. . . . Therefore glorify God in your body,
and in your spirit, which are God's.
1 Corinthians 6:19–20 kjv

∞

We may feel as though our bodies have failed us terribly—but they deserve our love and care now more than ever. Notice all that our bodies can still do. When we stop to think, we see that the mere ability to see and smell, taste and touch is wonderful and miraculous.

The Bible makes clear that God sends both physical and spiritual blessings into our lives. He wants our lives to be healthy—emotionally, physically, spiritually. We tend to separate the spiritual world from the physical one, but the Bible shows us a perspective where each sort of blessing flows into all the others. As we are spiritually blessed, our physical lives will be blessed as well. God loves our entire being, including our bodies!

Lord of the universe, You made all the delicate, inner parts of my body and knit me together in my mother's womb. Thank You for making me so wonderfully complex! Your workmanship is marvelous—how well I know it. You watched me as I was being formed in utter seclusion, as I was woven together in the dark of the womb. You saw me before I was born. Every day of my life was recorded in Your book. Every moment was laid out before a single day had passed. How precious are Your thoughts about me, O God. They cannot be numbered! I can't even count them; they outnumber the grains of sand! I fall asleep—and when I wake up, You are still with me! (Psalm 139:13–18).

My body is Your Spirit's sanctuary, Jesus. Your Spirit lives inside me! You have chosen my flesh and blood as the place from which You shine. And not only that—You died on the cross so that nothing would stand in the way of Your Spirit living within me. When I consider all that, I realize how much my body deserves my care. Why would I want anything to dim Your Spirit's light?

Remind me, loving God, that caring for my body is also spiritual discipline. It's not just about wanting to look good so I can impress others. You created my body. Jesus died for it. The Holy Spirit lives in it. It's connected to Christ. And one day it will be resurrected!

I will bless You, Lord, at all times; Your praise shall continually be in my mouth. I sought You, and You answered me and delivered me from all my fears. I look to You and become radiant; You make my face shine with health and joy. I cried out to You, and You heard me and delivered me from all my trouble. Your angels camped around me; You delivered me. And now, I taste life and see how good You are! I am physically blessed because I took refuge in You when I was weak. I don't lack anything, because You give me everything good that I need (Psalm 34:1, 3–10).

∞

Remind me, Lord, that caring for my body is also a way to worship You. Whatever I do, in word or deed, may I do everything in Your name, Lord Jesus, giving thanks to God the Father through You (Colossians 3:17).

God's Promises

For no matter how many promises God has made,
they are "Yes" in Christ. And so through him
the "Amen" is spoken by us to the glory of God.
2 CORINTHIANS 1:20 NIV

∞

A promise is a declaration about the future.
It's a commitment to do something, a statement
of a fact that has not yet come to pass. The Bible is
full of God's promises, His statements of all that
He will do for us. Even beauties of the natural
world—like rainbows—remind us that God has
promised to be faithful to His people, to give us
life rather than death, to shower us with blessings,
and to love us for eternity.

When cancer strikes our lives, we may feel as
though God's promises have been erased. We feel
as though we've fallen into a world where God's
love and blessing no longer reach us. But that's an
illusion. It's not the truth. Nothing can shake the
promises of God. Not even cancer.

With You on my side like this, God, how can I lose? If You didn't hesitate to put everything on the line for me, embracing my condition and exposing Yourself to the worst by sending Your own Son, is there anything else You wouldn't gladly and freely do for me? The One who died for me—who was raised to life for me!—is in Your presence at this very moment sticking up for me. And so I'm absolutely convinced that nothing—nothing living or dead, angelic or demonic, today or tomorrow, high or low, thinkable or unthinkable— absolutely *nothing* can get between me and Your love because of the way that Jesus my Master has embraced me (Romans 8:31–39 MSG).

Help me, Lord, be more like Abraham, who never wavered in believing Your promise. In fact, his faith grew stronger, and in this he brought glory to You (Romans 4:20). Make my faith stronger, too, so that I can give more glory to You.

God, You promised Abraham that You would bless him, make his name great, and make him a blessing to the world for generations to come (Genesis 12:2–3). Thank You that because I belong to Christ, I am a true child of Abraham. I am his heir, and Your promise to Abraham belongs to me (Galatians 3:29).

I saw You, Lord, always before me. Because
You are at my right hand, I will not be shaken.
Therefore my heart is glad and my tongue
rejoices; my body also will rest in hope,
because You have promised You won't abandon
me to the realm of the dead. You call me holy and
promise that I will not see death's decay. You have
made known to me the paths of life; You will fill
me with joy in Your presence. Thank You that You
have given me the gift of the Holy Spirit. Thank
You that Your promise is for me—and for my
children, for my grandchildren, and for all those
who are yet to be born (Acts 2:25–28, 38–39).

God, just when I thought I would never be able to praise You again, You put a new heart in me and gave me a new spirit. You took away my heart of stone and brought me back to life. And now You promise that You put Your Spirit within me and lead me in Your path, showing me the way to go (Ezekiel 36:26–27).

Now salvation and strength and the kingdom of God have come into my life, Lord, and the power of Christ, for You have cast down all that accused me and made me feel less. You have promised to overcome all death by the blood of the Lamb—and now I will love You more than life itself (Revelation 12:10–11).

Thank You, dear God, that You have promised
to always be my refuge in times of trouble.
Teach me to know Your name and put my trust
in You, because You have promised never to
forsake those who seek You (Psalm 9:9–10).

I know, heavenly Father, that mountains could
crumble—the worst could happen and everything
in my life could seem to fall apart—and even
then, You have promised that Your kindness will
never leave me. Your promise of peace will never
be taken away from me (Isaiah 54:10).

Thank You, Lord, that Your mercy is from
everlasting to everlasting—and that You
have promised to bless my children and my
children's children (Psalm 103:17). Your
promises give me strength to face the future.

Physical Healing

The LORD protects and preserves them—they are counted
among the blessed in the land—he does not give them over
to the desire of their foes. The LORD sustains them on their
sickbed and restores them from their bed of illness.

PSALM 41:2–3 NIV

∞

The Bible is full of stories about people who were physically healed by the Lord. These stories tell us that God's miraculous healing is possible in a physical sense. But the Bible always makes clear that ultimately, healing is a spiritual thing. God may use our physical illnesses—and even our physical deaths—to bring us to eternal wholeness.

So when we pray for physical healing, we need to surrender to God the method He chooses to use. Whatever happens, cancer will not have the final say!

Jesus, when You walked this earth, I know You
healed all sorts of diseases. People were always
reaching out to You, clamoring for Your healing.
Just the touch of Your robe sent Your healing
power flowing out to those who had been sick for
years. Jesus, I believe You are the same now as You
were then. You are filled with healing power.
If I could only touch Your robe!

∾

Jesus, I read in the Gospels how You went
around restoring people's vision, giving back the
ability to walk, allowing the deaf to hear, and
healing every illness You encountered. Even if I
can't destroy this cancer that's entered our lives,
I pray that nevertheless Your healing power
would work through me.

Thank You, heavenly Father, for doctors and medicine. Use them to bring healing. And thank You also that Your power is infinitely greater than any human wisdom or treatment. You are able to do immeasurably more than all we ask or imagine, according to Your power that is at work within us (Ephesians 3:20).

Jesus, You said that we could ask You for anything in Your name and You would do it (John 14:14). In the name of Jesus, I ask that You bring healing. Take away this cancer. Give wholeness and health. Deliver us from this enemy.

I know, Lord, that You don't always choose to heal those who are ill. Sometimes instead, You ask sick people to bear their infirmity. And yet even then, I believe You bring healing, the deepest healing that reaches to the depths of a person's soul and lasts until eternity. God, I ask You for that kind of healing. You know I wish I could be free from cancer, here, now, in this life. But give me the strength to bear it if instead You choose to heal me in other ways, ways I need even more. You know me better than I know myself. I'll trust Your love to do what's right for me and for my family.

Emotional Healing

He heals the brokenhearted and binds up their wounds.
PSALM 147:3 NIV

∽

*C*ancer leaves emotional wounds on everyone it touches. Our confidence in life is destroyed. Our relationships have changed. Our very sense of who we are has been broken.

But God has promised to heal our broken hearts. We may feel guilty letting others see our sadness and pain, but with God, we never need to pretend to be something we aren't. We don't need to impress Him with our spiritual maturity and mental health. Instead, we can come to Him honestly, with all our neediness, admitting just how weak we are. When we do, we let down the barriers that keep Him out of our hearts. We allow His grace to make us whole and healthy.

Thank You, Lord God, that You have promised that the Sun of Righteousness will rise with healing in His wings—and we will go free from all our sorrow and hurt, leaping with joy like calves let out to pasture. On the day when You take action, we will step over all that cancer has done in our lives, because You are the Lord of heaven's armies (Malachi 4:2; Psalm 80:19).

Jesus, I need to talk to someone who can help me with this emotional pain I'm feeling. Your Word promises that the words of a wise person will bring healing (Proverbs 12:18). Send me to the right person who can help me heal.

Jesus, I read in the Gospel that people came to hear You and be healed not only of their physical diseases but also from their emotional troubles. Whenever they touched You, Your power went out from You and brought healing to wounded minds (Luke 6:18–19). Lord, I need You to heal me, the same way You did those who could touch You with their physical hand. Help me feel Your touch.

Lord God, I know there is a time to plant and a time to uproot what is planted. . .a time to kill and a time to heal. . .a time to tear down and a time to build up. . .a time to weep and a time to laugh. . .a time to mourn and a time to dance (Ecclesiastes 3). I pray that this would be a time now for planting, for healing, for building up, for laughing, and for dancing.

Father God, heal my wounds. Give me emotional prosperity and true peace. Restore me and rebuild me emotionally so that I can bring joy, glory, and honor into the world. Let everyone see all the good You have done for me, all the peace and fullness I am experiencing now. I who was so desolate, who felt abandoned, will once more laugh out loud. I will sing and give thanks to You. I will tell everyone how good You are. Lord God, Your faithful love endures forever! After all that I have been through, You have brought me back to where I once was. You have made me whole and happy again (Jeremiah 33:6–11).

Spiritual Healing

He sent out his word and healed them,
snatching them from the door of death.
PSALM 107:20 NLT

∞

*C*ancer also leaves spiritual scars. Our faith has been tested in ways it never was before—and we may not yet feel able to trust God as we once did. That's okay! We need to learn *new* ways to trust Him. The old ways are over, and now it's time for new things.

God has a holistic perspective on health. He wants the entire package to be strong and fit. Health pours out of Him, a daily stream of grace that heals our spirits, even as it heals our bodies and minds.

Lord, make Yourself known to me anew so that I can know You as I never have before. Let me worship You in new ways and keep all my vows to You. Cancer struck me down, but now I ask that You use it to bring healing so that I will return to You even stronger than before. I know You will respond to me and heal me (Isaiah 19:21–22).

∞

I'm going back to You, Father. I feel as though You tore me to pieces—but I believe You will heal me. You injured me—but now You will bandage my wounds (Hosea 6:1).

∞

Jesus, You told Your disciples to heal the sick, telling them that Your kingdom of God was near to them (Luke 10:9). I ask that You send someone into my life who will help me see Your kingdom more clearly.

Dearest Lord, You have sent all my spiritual adversaries, every one of them, into captivity. That which plundered my spirit has been destroyed. Everything that preyed on me spiritually has fled. You are restoring me to health. You are healing my wounds. I felt like an outcast; I felt as though people must have been thinking that You didn't care about me anymore. But then You said to me, "Look! I will restore you. I will make you a new home. The ruin of your life will be rebuilt, better than before. You're going to live in a palace now! Everything will be put right within your spirit" (Jeremiah 30:16–18).

Father in heaven, You sustained me on my
sickbed. You restored me to physical health.
Now I ask You to send out Your grace and
heal my soul as well (Psalm 41:3–4).

I have no faith left, Lord—but
You promise to heal my faithlessness.
Your love knows no bounds (Hosea 14:4).

O God, be with my loved one who has suffered
so much. Do not let her be spiritually dead, now
that she has come through this terrible ordeal.
Don't let him be like a stillborn baby who didn't
survive its birth. O God, bring spiritual healing,
I pray! (Numbers 12:12–13).

Peace

*You will experience God's peace, which exceeds
anything we can understand. His peace will guard
your hearts and minds as you live in Christ Jesus.*
PHILIPPIANS 4:7 NLT

∞

The Hebrew word that is translated "peace"
is actually *shalom*. It's a word that is rich with
significance in the Hebrew language, with many
shades of meaning that add greater depth to our
usual concept of peace as simply the absence of
conflict. These meanings include completeness,
prosperity, safety, contentment, health, rest,
comfort, ease, and soundness. This is the sort of
peace that God promises will guard our hearts
and minds.

Jesus said, "I have told you these things, so
that in me you may have peace. In this world you
will have trouble. But take heart! I have overcome
the world" (John 16:33 NIV). Trust Him to be
the guardian of your mind and of your life. Allow
Him to create shalom even in the midst of cancer!

Jesus, thank You for coming to earth and sharing our human experiences. I know that in You I can find peace. In this world, I have run into hard times—but I will take heart, for I know You have overcome the world (John 16:33).

∽

Lord, help our family to pray the serenity prayer: "Grant us the serenity to accept the things we cannot change, the courage to change the things we can, and the wisdom to know the difference."

∽

Thank You, Jesus, that You have given me Your peace. I know Your peace is not like anything the world has to offer me. Because of You, I will not let my heart be troubled, neither will I let it be afraid (John 14:27).

Jesus, help me to rejoice, even now. Remind me to aim for perfect harmony with others. Even in this difficult time, may we encourage one another, be of one mind, and live in peace. Thank You that Your own Spirit of love and peace will be with us (2 Corinthians 13:11).

∾

Peace seems so far away sometimes, beloved Friend. It's not something I can work up in my heart on my own, no matter how hard I try. Instead, I know it's one of Your gifts of grace.

∾

Teach me to turn to You when I need peace. Jesus, thank You that even when we feel far away from You, You are still sending us Your message of peace, just as much as when we feel near to You. Thank You that through You we have access to the Father by one Spirit (Ephesians 2:17–18).

Your wisdom, God, is first of all pure, then peaceable, gentle, accommodating, full of mercy and good fruit, impartial, and sincere. Make me more like You, I pray. Help me to be a peacemaker who sows in peace during this time of sickness so that I will reap the fruit of righteousness (James 3:17–18).

I know, Lord, that some emotions nourish me and bring me closer to You—while I need to quickly drop others into Your hands as soon as they enter my heart. Teach me to cultivate and seek out that which brings peace. May I get better at letting go of my negative feelings as quickly as I can, releasing them to You. I know that if I cling to these dark feelings, they will reproduce worse than cancer cells do, blocking the healthy flow of grace into my life.

Christ, may Your peace rule in our hearts.
We know we are all members of Your body,
called to live in peace with each other,
now more than ever (Colossians 3:15).

∞

May Your peace, Lord Jesus, control my emotions,
my doubts, my worries. In fact, may peace control
my entire life. Help me live Your peace during
these days and through all that lies ahead.

∞

Beloved Friend, I want to focus my attention
on You. Remind me to give You all my worries,
one by one, every day. If I do, I know You will do
Your part—You will keep my heart at peace.

Hope

But you, LORD, are a shield around me, my glory, the One
who lifts my head high. I call out to the LORD, and he
answers me from his holy mountain. I lie down and sleep;
I wake again, because the LORD sustains me. I will not
fear though tens of thousands assail me on every side.
PSALM 3:3–6 NIV

∞

*H*ope is an attitude, not an emotion. It
means putting our whole heart into relying on
God. It means keeping our eyes focused on Him,
no matter what, waiting for Him to reveal Himself in our lives. God never disappoints those who
passionately wait for His help, who diligently seek
His grace.

When facing cancer, however, hope may
seem to take more courage than we can muster.
There is so much unknown in our lives, so much
that seems threatening. Like an animal caught
in the headlights of oncoming doom, we stand
frozen, helpless. But God is there in the darkness.
He will go with us each step of the way. Our
hope is in Him.

Lord, I put my hope in You,
for Your love never fails (Psalm 130:7).

∞

Thank You, God, that You have plans for me—
plans to bless me and prosper me. I know that
Your plans are often not the same as mine. But
You know what the future holds, and I trust You.

∞

"I look behind me and you're there, then up
ahead and you're there, too—your reassuring
presence, coming and going. This is too much,
too wonderful—I can't take it all in!"
(Psalm 139:5–6 MSG).

Lord, I feel as though I can't make it through one more day—or even one more minute. I can't endure any more. Help me have a hope that's big enough to just get me through the next minute. . .and then the one after that. Inch by inch, minute by minute, give me the hope I need to keep moving forward.

Jesus, You promised to never leave me or forsake me. Because of You, I have hope. I know this hope will never be put to shame.

Remind me, Jesus, that hope doesn't mean I run ahead of You. Only You know the future. And You are already there, waiting for me.

Thank You, God, that no matter what happens, You have given me the hope of eternal life. Thank You that You cannot lie—and You have given us this hope as a promise even before time began (Titus 1:2).

Father, make me like the Proverbs 31 woman— clothed with strength and dignity, able to laugh without fear of the future (Proverbs 31:25). Clothe me with Your strength and dignity, I pray. Make me whole, full of Your grace. I anticipate the future, knowing that You will take care of the details as I trust You to be the foundation of my life.

Lord Jesus, I know that I can love others better
when I put my hope in You. Love springs out
from the hope that You have stored up for me
in heaven, the same hope that I already possess
now through Your Good News. This is the Good
News that is bearing fruit in my life, and it keeps
on growing, just as it has since the very beginning,
because of Your grace (Colossians 1:4–6).

Christ Jesus, I'm waiting with blessed hope
for Your glorious appearance! You are my Savior,
the one who gave Yourself for me to redeem me
and make me whole (Titus 2:13–14).

I'm relying on You, loving God, to fulfill
my hopes—not the way I want them fulfilled,
but in ways I never could have expected.

Joy

Consider it pure joy, my brothers and sisters, whenever
you face trials of many kinds, because you know that
the testing of your faith produces perseverance.
JAMES 1:2–3 NIV

∞

*O*ne of the spiritual blessings God gives us is
joy—and all His other blessings increase that joy.
Joy is like a spring of water that keeps spilling
into our lives. Just when we think the spring has
run dry, when we feel as though we'll never feel
joy again, joy wells up. At first, it may just be a
tiny trickle—but then it grows into a rushing
stream that fills our hearts once more. In the
midst of sickness and fear and weakness, God still
blesses us with joy. Even cancer can't limit Him!

Jesus, help me see the joy hidden within this difficult time. I know that this testing of my faith will help me develop the ability to persevere—and that ability in turn will allow me to grow up in You and become complete, not lacking anything (James 1:2–4).

∞

May Your joy, Lord,
be my strength (Nehemiah 8:10).

∞

I know, Father, that You are not a God of sighing and gloom. I know You are waiting to share Your joy with me. Help me open myself to receive it.

Even when I feel lost in darkness, loving Lord, somehow Your joy catches up with me, like a surprise gift from someone I love. Thank You.

I know You are longing to give me the joy of Your presence. Remind me to seek You.

You are at work in my life. Your Spirit is moving and acting in amazing ways. The Creator of the world is working on my behalf—so why am I so filled with gloom? How can I help but laugh and sing when You have already triumphed over the forces of darkness?

My joy depends only on You, God. Help me realize that, so that I'll no longer worry so much about losing or gaining life's other blessings.

∞

Your Word tells me that a happy heart is like good medicine but a broken spirit will drain my strength (Proverbs 17:22). Give me a happy heart!

∞

You know that I function better when I'm happy, dear Lord. Discouragement and sadness sap my physical, emotional, and spiritual strength. It's like trying to work while carrying a heavy load on my back: it slows me down and makes everything harder. Heal my sadness, I pray. Send out Your grace to make me strong and happy.

Here's the surprising lesson cancer has taught me, Lord: when troubles come my way, I can consider it an opportunity for great joy (James 1:2).

Keep me always in Your love, Jesus, just as You kept Yourself always in Your Father's love. Then Your joy will be in me, and my joy will be complete. Remind me that the way to have this joy is by loving You and loving others (John 15:10–12).

You have ransomed me out of cancer, Lord, and now I can come to You with shouts of everlasting joy. All my sorrow and sighing will flee away (Isaiah 35:10).

Love

Love never gives up. . . . Always looks for the best, never looks back, but keeps going to the end. Love never dies.
1 CORINTHIANS 13:4–8 MSG

∞

We usually think of these verses as a description of how we should love others (which of course they are). But these familiar words also describe how God loves us. He never gives up on us. He doesn't worry about what we did in the past but always focuses on what's ahead. His love never wears out. Like the Energizer Bunny, it just keeps going. . .and going.

The Creator of the universe loves us—and His love is unconditional and limitless. We can never wear out His love. Even as we face all the pain and fear of cancer, we can know we are utterly and completely loved, no matter what, forever and ever.

Without Your love, Lord, my heart would be sad and lonely. Thank You that there will never be a moment of my life when I am not loved by You.

All Your blessings, Father God, both spiritual and physical, are wrapped up in Your love. Because You love me, You will never stop blessing me. Even now, as my family faces cancer, Your love never fails.

Jesus, You were the love of God walking on earth. You are the ultimate expression of divine love. Be real to me, I pray, so that I may know God's love, through all that lies ahead.

I know that my fears about the future say that
I still don't trust Your love, Lord Jesus. Send
Your perfect love, I pray, to drive out all my fear.
Teach me how to love as You first loved me
(1 John 4:18–19).

Thank You, heavenly Lord, that there is
nothing I need to do to deserve Your love.
I don't have to earn it. I don't have to be
lovable for You to love me!

God, I'm coming to know Your love because
it's touched me personally. The more I experience
it, the more I trust You. Now I'm starting to
depend on that love, knowing that You will
never jerk it out from under me. How could
You, when Your very nature is love?

Your unfailing love, O Lord, is as vast
as the heavens. Your faithfulness reaches
beyond the clouds (Psalm 36:5).

Put me like a seal over Your heart, dear God, like a
seal on Your arm. For love is as strong as death—
it's Your flame that nothing can quench, even
cancer! Nothing in this world is worth as much
to me as Your love (Song of Solomon 8:6–7).

Through all that has happened, I have come
to know and to believe the love that You have
for me, dearest Lord. You are love, and when
I abide in love, I abide in You—and You
abide in me (John 15:4).

Since You loved me so much, now I also ought to love others. I can't see You, God, but when I love others, You live in me, and Your love is made perfect in me. This is the only way I can know for sure that I'm living in You—if Your love pours through me out into the world. You have given me Your Spirit of love (1 John 4:11–13).

∞

Remind me, dear Jesus, that You have called me to share Your love with others. Make me a portrait of Your love. Use my hands, my feet, my words, my smile to show everyone I meet that You are real. Remind me that I still live because You want me to carry out Your work of love. Be visible through me, I pray.

Life

I am come that they might have life,
and that they might have it more abundantly.
JOHN 10:10 KJV

∞

ancer doesn't have to make our lives narrow
and restricted. That's not the way God wants us to
live. He sends His grace into our lives abundantly
so that our lives can be full of blessing. Even as
cancer looms over us, we can be assured that God
has promised us a full, rich life, a life that will
never end.

Jesus came to this earth so that our fears
about death could be put to rest. He has promised
us that He will not only bless us in this life, but
He has also prepared a place for us in the life
to come—and when we die, we will hear His
voice welcoming us into eternal life, a life more
abundant than we can imagine now.

God, I'm trying to accept what lies ahead.
But I don't want to face death. I'm glad that
Your Son felt the same way about it. He prayed
for a way around death, if there was any way
possible. He understands what I feel.

I'm glad, Lord, that Your scripture refers to
death as the "last enemy." I like knowing that
You and I are in this together, fighting this
battle together. And I know You will win!
You created me to live forever.

Thank You, dear Jesus, that I don't need to worry
about the future. No matter how frightening the
path ahead may seem, You have plans for me,
plans for good and not for disaster, to give me a
rich life that's filled with hope (Jeremiah 29:11).

Father, I know You want me to be healthy—
not just physically but emotionally, intellectually,
and spiritually as well. You want to fill my
life full of all the things I truly need. The life
You give to me isn't dry and empty and barren.
Instead, it is lush and full of delicious things that
will nourish me. Right now, I feel as though
I'm crossing a desert—but I know You will give
what I need to reach the next oasis.

∽

Even as I face cancer, You will show me
the way of life, dear God, granting me the
joy of Your presence and the pleasures of
living with You forever (Psalm 16:11).

Jesus, You said that if I want to follow You, I must deny myself and take up my cross. If cancer is the cross I have to bear, then give me strength to lift it. You also said that if all I care about is saving my life, I'm doomed in the end to lose it—but if I surrender my life to You, I'll save it. What good would it do me to be healthy, to have everything in life I want, if that meant I would lose You? The only way for me to possess life is to surrender it absolutely into Your hands.

As I let go of everything—even my life—
Your grace gives everything back to me,
transformed by Your love (Mark 8:35).

My life has always been a gift from You, Creator God. The blood that flows through my veins, the beat of my heart, and the breath in my lungs are Your gift to me, a mere token of the love You will shower on me in heaven.

∞

Since I am so richly loved, teach me to sing, even in the darkness, Lord.

∞

You have given me so much life, Father. Now let me give back to You and to those around me. I know that when I do, You will give me still more—so much that it has to be pressed down and shaken together to make room for more, and even then it will spill over. The amount of life I give away will only make room for more and more of Your life to be poured into me (Luke 6:38).

Let my heart keep Your commandments,
heavenly Lord, and You will give me life and
peace. Don't let Your kindness and truth leave me.
Bind them around my neck; write them on the
tablet of my heart (Proverbs 3:1–3).

∞

When I live in Your shelter, Most High One,
I find rest and life in Your shadow. You are my
only refuge, my only place of safety. You are my
God, and I trust You, for You have rescued me
from cancer's trap; You have protected me from
this deadly disease. You have covered me with
Your feathers and sheltered me with Your wings
so that I could live in You (Psalm 91:1–4).

I don't need to be afraid, Almighty One, of the fears that come in the night. Even if everyone around me is dying, I know that You are still my refuge and shelter. No evil will conquer me, no disease can destroy my home, for Your angels are protecting us. You have promised to rescue me; You have promised to answer when I call and to be with me through this time of trouble. And then You promise me even more—for You will honor me and give me a full life (Psalm 91:14–16).

What can I say, Lord Jesus? If You are for me, what can ever come against me? Since You gave up Your own life on my behalf, I can be confident You will give me everything else. You died for me—and then You came back to life for me so that You could share eternal life with me. Nothing can separate me from Your love! (Romans 8:31–39).